PRAISE FOR *7-DAY DETOX MIRACLE*

"An unfortunate reality of modern life is our high level of toxic exposure. Environmental pollution from industrial waste, build up of metabolic poisons due to nutritional deficiencies, antibiotic-induced abnormal bacteria in the gut, all add to increased toxicity and decreased health. The guidance and wisdom offered by Doctors Bennett and Barrie provide a welcome pathway to detoxification and restored vitality."

—Joseph E. Pizzorno Jr., N.D.,
president, Bastyr University and author of *Total Wellness*

"Physicians will lose their fear of the process after reading this book for they will understand it better. They will be able to treat their patients who are following detox programs recommended by their naturopaths more effectively. This is a valuable book. I know detoxification programs work for I have witnessed this over the past thirty years."

—Abram Hoffer, Ph.D., M.D., author of *Smart Nutrients*

"This book is an excellent 'how to and why' regarding environmental toxicity and detoxification. It is a valuable addition to the library of all clinicians and a clearly written guide for patients."

—Mitchell V. Kaminski Jr., M.D.

7-DAY DETOX MIRACLE

Revitalize Your Mind and Body with This Safe and Effective Life-Enhancing Program

REVISED 2ND EDITION

PETER BENNETT, N.D.
STEPHEN BARRIE, N.D.
SARA FAYE

 THREE RIVERS PRESS • NEW YORK

Published by Three Rivers Press, New York, New York. Member of the Crown Publishing Group, a division of Random House, Inc.
www.crownpublishing.com

THREE RIVERS PRESS and the Tugboat design are registered trademarks of Random House, Inc.

Originally published by Prima Publishing, Roseville, California, in 2001.

Interior graphics by Paula Bishop

EcoTox is a registered trademark of Peter Bennett, N.D., and Stephen Barrie, N.D.

Printed in the United States of America

Library of Congress Cataloging-in-Publication Data

Bennett, Peter, N.D.
    7-day detox miracle : revitalize your mind and body with this safe and effective life-enhancing program / Peter Bennett, Stephen Barrie, Sara Faye—2nd ed.
      p.   cm.
    Includes bibliographical references and index.
    1. Detoxification (Health). I. Title: Seven-day detox miracle. II. Barrie, Stephen. III. Faye, Sara. IV. Title.

RA784.5 .B46 2001
613—dc21   2001021765

ISBN 0-7615-3097-5

10 9 8 7 6

Second Edition

To all of our teachers
who imparted the importance
of personal effort and self-motivation
in the pursuit of Knowledge

CONTENTS

FOREWORD

The term "detoxification" means many things to different people. To the doctor specializing in toxicology it means the treatment for patients suffering from drug and chemical overdose, for the pharmacologist it means the mechanism by which the body metabolizes pharmaceutical substances and eliminates them from the body, for the environmental scientist it means the way that substances in the environment are decontaminated, for the chemically dependent person it means a treatment program designed to rid them of their drug addiction. In the context of the book *7-Day Detox Miracle* by Drs. Peter Bennett and Stephen Barrie, both naturopathic physicians of international distinction, it means the process whereby people who have chronic health complaints due to the low grade "poisoning" of their metabolism. As is eloquently described in this book, this low grade "poisoning" is something that happens to many of us as we accumulate toxins from a polluted environment, lifestyle habits such as smoking, excess alcohol and caffeine consumption, faulty diet, medications, stress, and too little activity.

What makes *7-Day Detox Miracle* such an important book is that it represents the clinical wisdom and experience of two doctors who have successfully practiced natural medicine over the past fifteen years that includes the use of science-based detoxification programs. Their clinical experience in the use of the approach described in *7-Day Detox Miracle* makes this book much more than a theoretical and interesting approach to improving health. Rather it is a tried and proven program for people who are looking for a way to get rid of chronic health complaints such as fatigue, low energy, digestive complaints, muscle aches and pains, and a myriad of other aggravating symptoms.

As a nutritional biochemist who has been involved in research focused on the better understanding of how nutrition influences the body's detoxification process, I found Drs. Bennett and Barrie's book to represent a significant contribution to making this concept more accessible to the average person who can benefit from its application.

Biochemists often speak in very specialized jargon that makes their message hard to understand. Drs. Bennett and Barrie have made a major accomplishment by weaving together in understandable terms the basics of the physiological and biochemical processes of detoxification with their clinical experience in how this information can be used for improved health. The most amazing distinction of the book is that they have done this without compromising the integrity of either the science or the easy reading style of the book.

By using case histories and clinical experiences the story of the *7-Day Detox Miracle* unfolds. From our experience at our Functional Medicine Research Center, our clinical staff has found that a nutritionally supported detoxification program can help improve the health and functional vitality of many people who are "walking tired."

Although no single program is successful for all people, *7-Day Detox Miracle* does provide a very well-formulated and clinically evaluated approach to accessing the power of our own body's detoxification and recuperative abilities. It is interesting that nutritionally based detoxification is not considered a standard approach in medicine even though it has been demonstrated to reduce migraine headaches, improve the muscle pain of fibromyalgia, and improve sleep in many studies. This may be a result of the fact that medicine today is based upon the presumption that "don't fix it until it's broken." A person may not be sick enough yet to be seen as "broken" during this age of managed care, but rather may be suffering from a significant reduction in their quality of life due to chronic symptoms for which *7-Day Detox Miracle* could be of great value.

I am very pleased that Drs. Bennett and Barrie have written this very helpful book that will make the power of nutritionally based detoxification more accessible to countless people.

Jeffrey S. Bland, Ph.D., President,
Institute for Functional Medicine

ACKNOWLEDGMENTS

No book can be written without the enthusiasm and contribution of other people. The librarians at Healthcomm were very helpful finding and sending research material; John Furlong, N.D., was very focused in providing salient research; Jeff Bland, Ph.D., was inspiring in his vast knowledge of the subject; Paula Bishop was amazing at generating graphics with no time and very little guidance; Brad Rachman, D.C., was a wonderful source of ideas and organization; and Jennifer Risden at Prima successfully navigated a complex edit.

PREFACE TO 2ND EDITION

After interviewing hundreds of people who tried this program and after using this book in my clinic with all our patients, I have made several revisions, updates, and additions in this new edition. Happily, I found that most people found the first edition easy to use and the program effective. Some even said that it changed their lives by reversing long-standing health problems and giving a new sense of control. We were very pleased to hear that many people who used this program lost the weight that they needed to and that they kept that weight off.

A wonderful response to the first edition was that many medical doctors recommended this program to their patients. I had calls from people who had beneficial results after their doctors told them to try detoxification. This confirms that some physicians are integrating alternative strategies into their conventional health care. Appendix D provides information on referrals to medical doctors who will supervise you in this program.

May everyone enjoy good health,
Peter Bennett

PREFACE

Detoxification is a process of cleaning, nourishing, and resting the body, from the inside out. It works because it addresses the needs of individual cells, the smallest units of human life. Disturbed cellular function is the basis of disease, poor health, and lowered physical and mental performance. This medical strategy is commonly employed by doctors of naturopathic medicine who understand organ systems and organ function at the cellular level. The approach expresses a "global," inclusive whole-body perspective. It is a form of medicine that replaces the reductionist model of treating single body parts or organs separately with an ecosystem view of human health, a synergistic web of mind, body, and spirit.

Detoxification medicine is an ancient concept that appears as part of many healthcare systems around the world. In Europe, detoxification is considered a valid medical therapy and is offered at many health spas, under the supervision of mainstream medical doctors. As a treatment, detoxification is more important today than ever before because, in addition to the health problems humans have been experiencing for thousands of years, we are now exposed to a huge variety of environmental poisons. The seven-day detoxification plan described in this book offers you these time-tested detoxification techniques in a simple do-it-yourself form developed to deal with new environmental toxicity syndromes. This type of detoxification should not be confused with the process of helping people break free of their dependency on alcohol and drugs.

We call our method the EcoTox program. It's built on the core concepts of resting the immune and detoxification systems and the organs of the digestive tract while at the same time promoting elimination. We were taught about the validity of detoxification medicine from doctors who have been using it successfully with their patients for over 50 years. Scientific research supports our own years of clinical experience. This is a safe and effective method to enhance the body's own self-healing mechanisms. If you're sick, detoxification can help. If you're well, it will make you feel even better. That's why we refer to the therapy as the seven-day miracle. It can cure many chronic health problems and alleviate the symptoms of others; protect the body from disease; restore and enhance vitality; allow you to look your best; and ensure your ability to maintain optimum health.

CHAPTER 1

Health and Detoxification

- The EcoTox Detoxification Program
- What Is Health?

- The Defense Mechanism Model and Detoxification Medicine
- Take Charge of Your Health

W hy do we lose our health? What causes certain organs and systems to change, to move away from normal, healthy function? These are questions that concern all of us. Susceptibility to disease and illness is the result of inherited weaknesses, environmental exposures, and lifestyle stresses. These obstacles create changes in the cells of the body and affect our struggle to attain and maintain good health.

A certain wisdom is built into every life form, each of which is highly sensible and organized. Each life form is a resilient ecosystem reflecting a larger cosmic intelligence. Humans, as they have evolved, have adapted to their environment over the past five million years. Until modern times, the stresses of everyday life were fairly constant and predictable. These consisted of hunger, thirst, cold, heat, and bacteria-based diseases.

Enter the new millennium. Everything about our environment has changed radically. Now we must cope with new sources of toxins. Since the industrial revolution, thousands of chemical compounds never seen before have been introduced into the environment. We're constantly exposed to multiple toxins found in our medications, food, water, and air. Each one poses serious health risks, and little is known about how they interact and the ways in which two or more toxins, acting together, impact our health. We have mercury fillings in our teeth and ecosystem, anaerobic bacteria in our root canals, abnormal (bacterial) flora in our guts from antibiotics, lead in our bones from the years when leaded gasoline fueled our cars and machines, and drugs in our bloodstream that throw liver metabolism out of balance. This proliferation of toxic sources demands, more than ever, that we consider detoxifying our bodies. Toxins that damage the cells of the body are invisible and insidious. They break down the "invironment" of all body systems at the cellular level. This happens slowly, day by day, year after year, and so is difficult to detect until the actual onset of disease.

Disease from toxicity is caused by the presence of biochemicals that poison the blood and spread via the circulatory system. As a result, cells and tissues are literally "swimming" in a contaminated environment. Detoxification is a treatment regimen that cleans the blood and removes toxins from the body.

Detoxification enzyme systems in our cells have evolved that allow us to survive as we come into contact with thousands of toxic substances every day. They provide us with the natural ability to transform poisons into nontoxic elements that the body can reuse or eliminate. This is a type of biological alchemy, a mysterious and wonderful process that takes place on a daily basis—in our sleep and while we work. We aren't even aware of the miracle that's going on in every cell of our body.

Since this book is a primer in detoxification, it is important to distinguish three main areas of detoxification medicine:

1. Heavy metal exposure (lead, mercury, and cadmium)

2. Pesticide and organic solvent residues (PCBs) stored in human fat tissue

3. Altered intestinal ecology

Each of these areas of detoxification (metals, pesticides, and gut ecology) has its own medical literature base, and generally these areas are not thought of as related. The cells in our bodies don't know that medical science considers these different areas of toxicology as separate. Our cells are bathed in an environment that mixes all three classes of toxins, which have the potential to cause disease in our bodies.

It has been through our clinical experience, not medical research, that we have understood the importance of a multiple-intervention detoxification therapy. A complete detoxification therapy should include (1) dietary therapy to reduce intestinal membrane inflammation and altered bowel flora, (2) nutritional supplements to increase Phase 1 and Phase 2 liver detoxification and stimulate bile flow, and (3) sauna therapy to enhance the reduction of fat-stored pesticide metabolites.

This multiple-intervention therapy stimulates the function of the liver, spleen, lymphatics, and digestive tract (reticuloendothelial system). Medical science has described this system as a filtering organ that provides very important immune and regulatory functions. To date, there are no medical textbooks, surgical procedures, or drugs that create a process to enhance the function of this extremely important "blood cleaning" organ system. The work by naturopathic physicians and other holistic medical practitioners who use detoxification therapy represents an attempt to open up the concept of a medical specialty in "reticuloendotheliology" and a need for more research and clinical application of therapies that work with the reticuloendothelial system. The complete mechanisms by which detoxification therapy works need to be fully uncovered by medical science.

Detoxification is not a new way of healing. It isn't a New Age concept floated out on a weekend workshop, it isn't the latest healing fad flown in from the East, and it isn't a process that's foreign to your cells. Rather, detoxification is the way in which the body heals itself—an internal cleansing process that takes place continuously. It is truly miraculous. Detoxification medicine is a medical strategy for eliminating the obstacles to health. Just as antibiotics are a strategy for ridding the body of harmful bacteria, detoxification medicine is used to remove the toxins that disturb the cells' ability to function normally. At the same time, cells receive nutritional support to maximize their activity. This enhances the body's own self-healing mechanisms.

We're constantly exposed to multiple toxins found in our medications, food, water, and air. Each one poses serious health risks.

The toxin and the organism can be thought of as two samurai ready for battle. Both are biochemically alive and well trained. The contest is to see which is stronger. The strength of a toxin, or its toxicity, depends both on how effectively it blocks critical cell functions and on the cell's ability to deal with the toxin's life-blocking strength. Each cell's capacity to deal with toxins varies greatly, and many factors conspire to alter these variables. Inherited physical weaknesses, lifestyle stresses, and environmental exposure change a cell's capacity to break down toxins. This is what accounts for the fact that one person gets sick and another, subject to the same conditions, does not.

Research has shown that our ability to detoxify our internal environments bears a direct relationship to our susceptibility to disease. If your detoxification mechanisms are weak, you'll be more prone to early aging, heart disease, cancer, and chronic degenerative diseases. Both prevention and treatment depend on your capacity to detoxify. Detoxification protects the nervous, cardiovascular, and immune systems. By learning how to enhance your body's ability to detoxify, you'll be better able to stay healthy and feel young.

Using current medical research and traditional naturopathic detoxification therapies, we have put together a seven-day plan, which we'll refer to as the EcoTox detoxification program—a system of diet (with foods and supplements you can readily find at grocery or health food stores) and exercises and activities to stimulate circulation (which you can do at home alone or with a friend to give you a hand). This program as outlined here in this book helps you minimize your risk for disease as a result of toxicity syndromes and uses natural detoxification mechanisms to promote healing. Here are some relevant definitions to help you understand some important detoxification concepts.

Toxicology is the study of the effects of noxious or harmful substances on living organisms.

Biochemical toxicology is the science of biochemical mechanisms that transform molecules from toxic to nontoxic states.

Xenobiotics are chemicals or molecules that are foreign to biological systems.

The process of detoxification is the therapeutic biochemical, physiological, and nutritional approach to decreasing the impact of xenobiotics on the cellular physiology.

Toxicity describes the disturbing influences of a xenobiotic on cell physiology and the mechanisms or abilities of the body to deal with a poison.

The EcoTox Detoxification Program

The term *EcoTox* describes the overall concept of our approach to detoxification. *EcoTox* is a combination of the words *ecology* and *toxin*. Ecology is the science concerned with the relationships between organisms and their environments. In environmental studies, ecology is the study of the detrimental effects of modern civilization on the environment with a view toward preventing or reversing those effects through conservation.

Used together, ecology and toxin suggest a link among health, the environment, and the actions of toxins. As a word and a concept, *EcoTox* goes beyond the simple notion of detoxification, embodying a new definition of health equilibrium based on the weblike connections between the outer environment we live in and the inner environment of our bodies. It incorporates the core concepts of holistic medicine, preventive medicine, and wellness medicine and focuses on the need to bring harmony to our cellular biochemistry through detoxification methods. This approach to health care contributes to youthful vitality, longevity, and wellness, and it can alleviate chronic disease. Although our approach goes beyond just detoxification, keep in mind that whatever you can do to help your body detoxify and eliminate exposure to toxins may be of benefit. The guidelines

Case History

Alice was seventy-two years old and had been bothered by abdominal pain, obesity, and fatigue for several years. Her doctors diagnosed gall bladder disease and told her she needed surgery. She followed their instructions and although her gall bladder was removed, her pain and problems persisted. Her energy continued to decline despite the use of vitamins, prayers, and positive thinking.

After an initial evaluation, we placed Alice on our detoxification program with daily observation at our clinic. Initially her energy was low, and she experienced headaches and dizziness as her body adjusted to the change. After a few days, however, her complexion changed from its chronic pasty color to a healthy glow, her mind and memory cleared (helping to relieve her fatigue), and her abdominal pain completely disappeared.

We discovered her problem was rooted in what she ate. In all of her seventy-two years, she had never missed a meal, and she had overwhelmed her digestive system with too much food. In addition, she had irritated her intestinal tract by eating foods that we found she was allergic to. Like many people, Alice was unaware that if you have a sensitivity or allergy to certain foods, the reactions caused by exposure to them can have toxic consequences. Alice now avoids these foods, which were toxic to her system. She continues to lose weight while eating the foods that satisfy her and make her feel well.

that make up our detoxification strategy work by "turning on" and supporting the body's own mechanisms for managing and eliminating toxins and metabolic waste. We'll present these in detail in chapter 8.

No matter what disease or health problem you suffer from, detoxification medicine can help because it encourages vital organs and organ groups such as the brain, the kidneys, the liver, the cardiovascular system, and the immune system to function at full capacity and can even amplify their performance. Not everyone will experience relief from all their aches, pains, and problems in one week, but after seven days of stimulating cellular detoxification, many of those who use this program feel better. They report having more energy, improved digestion, and enhanced mental faculties.

This book gives you a blueprint for health. It is a program that can be individualized to your particular weaknesses to help prevent disease and cure chronic illness. We can't promise that everyone who's sick will be cured after following the program for seven days. But we can assure you that, at the very least, you'll be closer to wellness, with fewer, less troublesome symptoms and more internal strength to combat illness. You can apply the ideas outlined in this book and become your own health advocate by taking charge of your own wellness program. You could save hundreds or even thousands of dollars in medical expenses during your lifetime by using detoxification therapy.

Just as toxins are ravaging the environment around us, they are destroying the human body's internal biochemical and biomechanical atmosphere. To heal the damage they inflict, you need to intentionally re-create a normal, healthy, balanced internal ecology in your body. This is as profound and as thrilling as the restoration of a damaged ecosystem by conservation agencies. You're the conservation warden who watches over the ecology of your mind and body. Detoxification is the first phase of your personal restoration program.

What Is Health?

Everyone has different definitions of health and disease, and no single definition for either term fits all cultures, ages, and individuals. If you're twenty-five years old, your definition of health will likely have changed by the time you're seventy-five. Disease is a state in which certain cells in the body cannot perform the job they are meant to do. Symptoms are a sign that cells are damaged and function has been lost. So a good working definition of health is that it is proper cellular function expressed as optimum physical, mental, and emotional performance.

Conventional medical training programs focus mainly on pathology, drug and surgical therapies, and symptom management. The job of the physician and the medical-care delivery team is to take over where the body has failed. The body's ability to self-heal is generally not accounted for, an attitude that's reflected in the public's understanding of diagnosis, sickness, and health.

By learning how to enhance your body's ability to detoxify, you'll be better able to stay healthy and feel young.

Once you understand that your body is designed to regulate and repair itself, you'll be ready to look at health care in a new way. You'll never again be willing to settle for a therapeutic approach that focuses simply on naming your illness and suppressing your symptoms. Detoxification is the tool you can use to fight disease and promote health, strengthening your body cell by cell and revitalizing its ability to heal itself.

Mind–Body Health

A relationship exists between health, the activity of the mind, and toxins in the environment. Toxins affect the ways in which we think and feel, and thoughts and feelings affect the ways in which we process environmental toxins. It's a two-way street. Negative mental states—expressed as anxiety, panic, anger, depression, neurotic behavior, self-deprecation, self-destructive feelings and tendencies, and a weak will to live— can be triggered by conditions of toxicity, and they also hinder the ideal functioning of your built-in detoxification system. The brain produces hormones and substances in response to stressors, and these substances disrupt the body's delicate biochemical balance, changing the ways in which organs and systems operate. It's known, for example, that stress hormones slow down the activity of detoxification enzymes in the liver.

Mental and emotional strain contributes to almost every known disease: autoimmune disease, infectious disease from viruses or bacteria, cancer, and even skin diseases. All acute, chronic, and degenerative diseases are affected by one's mental and emotional state. Medical research has verified the effects of positive and negative thinking in heart disease and cancer, the leading causes of death in North America. For example, it has been established that even low levels of stress trigger the onset of angina. We also know that attitudes and emotional states are critical in fighting disease. The opposite is also true. Laughter, hope, acceptance, and the reduction of emotional and mental suffering speed the course of healing and decrease pain. If you can consistently visualize a state of wellness, you are more likely to achieve that state of wellness.

Therefore, to remain healthy every person should develop strategies for stress management and for maintaining a positive attitude, taking advantage of techniques such as therapy, support groups, and meditation. Every doctor's health care approach should reflect this scientific reality.

To get the most advantage from detoxification medicine, you must have a lifestyle and an outlook that support positive emotional states and that reduce negative emotions. We've included some techniques later in this book to help you.

The Defense Mechanism Model and Detoxification Medicine

The body has a natural defense mechanism that always attempts to protect the most important organs. This defense mechanism is not any single organ or structure in the body. Rather, it's the cumulative result of many internal systems, including the immune system and the brain, working in cooperation to set health priorities and shield critical organs from disease. The defense mechanism directs and controls the ways in which we fall ill and become well.

There is a useful model for understanding the effects of disease and the process of healing. As you can see in figure 1.1, as organisms, each of us is organized in a hierarchy. Tissues, organs, systems, and even states of mind are ranked according to each one's level of importance to the function of the whole. There are three "bodies": the physical, the emotional, and the mental. If you visualize a pyramid, the physical body is at the base, the emotional body is in the middle, and the mental body is at the top.

Within each of these "bodies" are five levels of priority. For the physical body, the skin and skeletal systems are the first, primary level, followed by the kidneys and genitals, the liver and the digestive system, the heart and lungs, and finally the brain and nervous system at the top. In the emotional body, worry comes first, followed by fear, anger, hysteria, and finally suicidal depression. The levels within the mental body are expressed as dullness and sloth, anxiety, cognitive dysfunction and memory loss, delusional states and dementia, and finally coma.

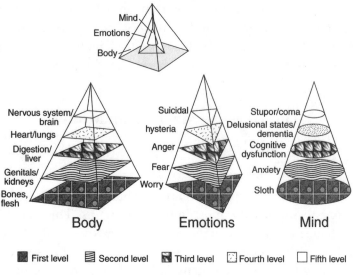

Figure 1.1

Each "body" (body, emotions, mind) contains five levels of priority.
The farther into a person's body-emotions-mind pyramid a disease enters,
the higher the degree of toxicity.

Disease tends to start at the base of the pyramid with the physical body, moving through each of its successive levels. If not stopped, the disease condition advances through the five levels of the emotional body and if unchecked continues through the levels of the mental body. Often, when only the symptoms of disease are treated rather than the disease itself, the condition is simply "pushed" to the next level of priority and farther up the hierarchy.

A disease that penetrates into a higher-ranked level indicates stronger shock and stress to the system and suggests that a weakness exists in the defense mechanism. The more toxic the patient, the deeper the penetration of symptoms into the hierarchy of the body. The greater the level of toxicity in the body, the more severe the disturbance in the defense mechanism and the longer detoxification therapy will need to be used. We heal from the top down, from the inside out, and from the most recent disease to the oldest. This concept was formulated by Constantine Herring, a renowned homeopath of the nineteenth century and is known as Herring's Law.

Figure 1.1 is applicable to you in that as you get better, your healing will move from deep levels of disease to more superficial levels. Mental symptoms of sloth or anxiety can be replaced with emotional symptoms of fear or worry. Emotional symptoms of anger can be replaced with physical symptoms of gallbladder pain or skin eruptions.

Improvement of one's health with detoxification is noticeable on a daily basis. Recovery is based on an individualized standard of evaluation that we call the three points of recovery: genetics, strength of disturbance, and interference.

Genetics

Human beings are not created biochemically alike. We inherit genetic traits that, to a large extent, determine our vulnerability to disease, our resistance to aging, and our capacity to handle environmental toxins. Inherited predispositions to disease might or might not manifest, depending on a variety of environmental factors. The deeper the inherited trait, the longer it takes to treat. A physician who takes a detailed family history will be better able to understand the nature of your health and the patterns that are likely to emerge as you get better.

Strength of Disturbance

The ability of a disease or a toxin to disrupt health depends both on its strength and on the strength of your body's defense mechanisms. If emotional pain or any physical or mental disturbance weakens your defenses, you become more vulnerable. The stronger the shock and the weaker your defenses, the more damage is done, and the longer is the required treatment time.

Interference

Interference with the body's natural ability to handle disease through the inappropriate application of therapies, such as drugs that put an additional burden on the body's detoxification mechanisms, can alter the timetable for recovery. When the body's natural healing mechanisms have been disturbed, the prognosis becomes more uncertain. Patients who have taken steroids, are on immunosuppressive drugs, or take certain prescribed medications on a daily basis generally require longer courses of detoxification treatment. In these cases, it's critical to take a "wait and see" approach. We are continually amazed when patients whom we didn't think we could help—because of medical histories that involved extensive medications and surgeries—fully recover.

Take Charge of Your Health

Those who practice mainstream medicine might be unaware or critical of the enormous body of medical literature that supports the safety, efficacy, and cost-effectiveness of detoxification medicine. Detoxification programs are the culmination of more than a hundred years of research and clinical delivery, and many gifted practitioners have contributed to the development of various approaches to such programs. These ideas have been embraced mainly by naturopathic physicians, but medical doctors, osteopaths, acupuncturists, and chiropractors have also used detoxification medicine with excellent results.

The ancient Indian and Chinese medical systems were built on the principles of detoxification. For centuries, physicians from different eras, countries, and cultures have seen the same thing: Allowing the body to detoxify can alleviate chronic disease and helps patients attain maximum wellness.

Unfortunately, timeless approaches to health care sometimes produce a knee-jerk response in highly trained physicians and specialists who equate it with snake oil and ignorance. The trend is to trust what is new and to ignore what was known in the preindustrial past. It's a classic case of throwing the baby out with the bath water.

If you are determined to get well and stay well, it's time to think for yourself and take the following steps.

1. Make your own decision on the basis of what you believe to be the best course of action for you.

2. Try to educate your family, friends, and health care providers about detoxification.

3. Find a physician who is able to help you with this system of care. In the appendix at the back of this book, you'll find information about how to locate a health care provider trained in detoxification medicine.

But remember, no doctor can help you if you won't help yourself. Many of our patients know that their habits and lifestyle are harmful to their health, but they're unwilling to change.

We try to help people understand what they need to do and why, but frequently they question our advice or hesitate to follow it. This is understandable, especially in light of the fact that their attitudes have been formed by medical literature and other sources that don't take into account the work of respected scientists and clinicians who function outside the boundaries of the medical mainstream. We explain that they've been getting their information from people who don't use the types of therapy that we do and who know little about the approach of naturopathic doctors and others who use so-called alternative therapies.

This book provides you with the information you need to start regaining and maintaining your health. If you feel good and have no symptoms, congratulations. However, before you decide that you don't need to clean house internally, remember that detoxification is the definitive concept in wellness medicine. It's an excellent way to prevent disease and protect your health. Common sense and medical physiology indicate that hardworking bodies need a rest and a tune-up every now and then. Regular downtime for every bodily system is the secret to maintaining vitality both now and in the future.

Once you understand that your body is designed to regulate and repair itself, you'll be ready to look at health care in a new way.

It can take years for symptoms to surface. Although you might not feel sick, your body may be holding off disease with all of its defense mechanisms. Eventually, the dam can break, and that's when illness appears. Even if you feel fine, consider a thorough evaluation to check your detoxification chemistry. The results might surprise you. Or, simply try the program, and see how much better you can feel.

This chapter is probably the most important in the book. When teaching patients to take charge of their health to recover it, they are always instructed to read this chapter

17

The Antibiotic Dilemma

Just as people are being forced to adapt to a changing environment, doctors must adapt to a new way of thinking. Use of antibiotics is a case in point. Antibiotics don't fight many infections, but doctors continue to use them. These drugs cause antibiotic resistance in bacteria and alter the delicate immune balance in the intestinal tract. It is important to save these drugs for those situations where they are indicated.

We saw a four-year-old boy who had been given thirty courses of antibiotics over three years for chronic ear infections. When a child is medicated like this, it creates a serious disturbance in the bowel flora and immune system. We were struck with chilling awareness that the drug solution that was supposed to have helped instead caused great harm. Studies have shown that children with recurrent ear infections are commonly allergic to certain foods, and antibiotics do nothing to treat the source of the problem: the allergic reactions to foods. In one study, children who did not receive antibiotics actually had fewer recurrences of ear infections than those who did. Keeping these points in mind, we identified the boy's food intolerances and eliminated those foods from his diet. After several months of detoxification to repair his intestinal tract and revive his immune system, the child had no further ear infections and thus no need for antibiotics.

first because it gives them a framework for thinking about their health. Because teaching a person how to think is more important than actually helping them, it is probably helpful to re-read this material several times.

Detoxification programs are the culmination of more than a hundred years of research and clinical delivery, and many gifted practitioners have contributed to various approaches.

Most people usually associate the word *detox* with programs to help those addicted to alcohol and drugs. But that is not what is meant by the term *detoxification medicine,* which is a very specialized kind of health care. It recognizes that the body has its own built-in healing system. Supporting that system by removing and eliminating toxins and supercharging every cell with healthy nutritional fuel is the natural way to treat and prevent disease. The first step is to realize that all of us are exposed to toxins every day, and some of us are more vulnerable to their harmful effects. It's a fact of life in our modern world. To protect your health, it's important to understand how toxins alter cellular activity.

CHAPTER 2

How Toxins Affect Your Health

- Cellular Basics
- Toxic Synergism
- Toxic Syndromes
- Signs of Toxicity
- Signs of Health

The most urgent question in human suffering is how to prevent disease. This question takes on a very personal significance when you realize that the choices you make each day form the foundation of your health, or lack thereof. Your lifestyle can foster the beginning of disease, which starts as a breakdown in the biochemistry of the body's cells, or further its spread into other tissues and organs. Toxins, both those that are man-made and those that the body manufactures, lead to this cellular breakdown if they are not removed from circulating blood and eliminated from the body.

The factors that influence your health and the bio-chemistry of your cells are complex, but a few basic points can help you understand them. Once you understand what your cells need to survive, you can begin to give them your personal care.

Cellular Basics

Nutritional medicine is the science of cellular health. Your body is made up of trillions of cells and the needs of each one of those cells are the same. When the needs of cells are not met, illness and sickness set in and we call this disease. When the needs of our trillions of cells are met on a daily basis, that is the beginning of good health (see figure 2.1) Each cell is perfectly designed to do the job it is assigned to do, and each cell is meant to work at full capacity. Diseases and poor health begin when individual cells are unable to do their work properly because their basic needs are not being met or something is inhibiting their function. A lack of nutrients, insufficient oxygen, poor waste removal, and the buildup of dangerous chemicals in the cells' environment inhibit cell function. Your task is to remove the obstacles that keep the cell from doing its work; this is the purpose of this three-part, seven-day detoxification program. First you identify the precise factors that block your health, then you learn how to repair the damage and stimulate your body to heal itself.

Eating an unhealthful diet and living an unhealthy lifestyle create an environment inside the body that disturbs the delicate balance necessary for high-performance cell functions. These factors, coupled with environmental pollution coming from outside the body, add to the body's usual detoxification duties—the regular removal and management of waste produced by normal cellular processes. This combined load can be too much for the body's machinery

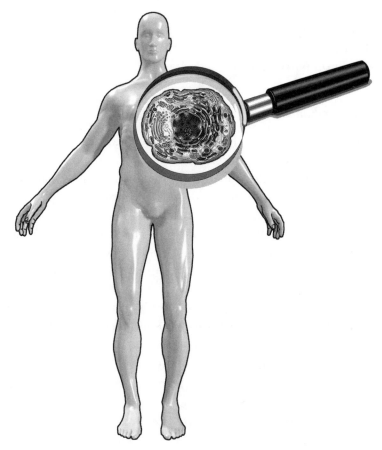

Figure 2.1

Your body is made of trillions of cells. In order to keep all your systems func-

tioning properly, you must take care that the needs of your cells are met.

to handle. When even further burdened by other factors like the excessive use of medications, heavy consumption of alcohol, and internal conditions such as intestinal permeability (also known as leaky gut syndrome), your body's systems react by slowing down, shutting down, or functioning erratically.

We can absorb only so many toxic stressors before cellular function and organ capacity begin to show signs of weakness and damage. This distress coincides with the onset of disease symptoms. Disease represents the weakening of the detoxification mechanisms inside the body. When this condition persists, health suffers.

Cellular Functioning

Poor health is not really caused by bacteria, viruses, or a failing organ. Rather, poor health results from poor cellular functioning that disrupts organ activity and allows bacteria and viruses to gain a foothold. At every moment, trillions of cells in your body are trying to survive. The problem is that cells encounter obstacles that don't allow them to work as they should. If we are conscious of this and take responsibility for supplying them with what they need, cells can survive, heal, and do their work.

The needs of cells are very simple. They are not greedy, needy, neurotic whiners. Each cell wants only three things: food (nutrients), a little conversation (the cell-to-cell communication that drives the metabolic machinery), and, perhaps most importantly, a clean house (proper elimination of toxins and waste products).

The cells' diet is made up of oxygen and about fifty different nutrients (see table 2.1). The circulatory and lymphatic systems remove accumulated waste from cells. Waste products come from the biochemical activity called metabolism that takes place inside the cell. The cell works hard: It "sweats" metabolic by-products and doesn't like to sit in its own muck, so it ships these by-products out via the bloodstream to the kidneys and the liver. There, they are processed and prepared for the final stage of elimination. When this doesn't happen, waste accumulates and the cell begins to poison itself. Most sick people become toxic because poisonous metabolic waste is being recycled back into their cells instead of being removed.

Table 2.1. *Food-Based Nutrients Critical to Cell Health (in order of importance)*

Water	***Trace Minerals***
Carbohydrates	Iron
Fiber	Copper
Essential Amino Acids	Iodine
Arginine	Manganese
Histidine	Chromium
Leucine	Zinc
Isoleucine	Fluorine
Lysine	Selenium
Methionine	Molybdenum
Phenylalanine	Tin
Threonine	Silicon
Tryptophan	Vanadium
Valine	Cobalt
Essential Fatty Acids	Nickel
Linoleic acid	Arsenic
Linolenic acid	***Water-Soluble Vitamins***
Arachidonic acid	Vitamin B_1 (thiamin)
Minerals	Vitamin B_2 (riboflavin)
Sodium	Vitamin B_3 (niacin)
Magnesium	Vitamin B_5 (pantothenic acid)
Phosphorous	Vitamin B_6 (pyridoxine)
Chlorine	Vitamin B_{12} (cyanocobalamin)
Potassium	Folic acid
Calcium	Biotin
Fat-Soluble Vitamins	Vitamin C (ascorbic acid)
Vitamin A (retinol)	
Vitamin D	
Vitamin E	
Vitamin K	

SOURCE: Adapted from The Kellogg Report.

Cellular Medicine

Those who practice cellular medicine, also referred to as detoxification medicine, address the body's needs at the cellular level. This "micro" approach has "macro" benefits. Evaluation focuses on the most fundamental level of dysfunction, and the root cause of a problem, rather than just its symptoms, is treated. This is very important in light of the fact that toxins affect our health by disturbing cell function, which can result in multiple organ involvement. In cellular medicine, each body part is considered in relation to all the others. In addition, each person reacts to toxins in a different way. So every case must be assessed individually.

First you identify the precise factors that block your health, then you learn how to repair the damage and stimulate your body to heal itself.

The practice of mainstream medicine is different. Medical doctors are trained to evaluate and treat organs and organ systems and to consider them as separate and distinctive health care specialties. There are cardiologists, neurologists, and gastroenterologists. When a patient consults this type of physician about his or her problems, the typical process is to try to match symptoms with disease complexes, conditions, and disorders familiar to the doctor in order to reach a diagnosis. Once the problem has been named, tests

Case History

Larry was told by his doctors that he had multiple sclerosis (MS). His overall weakness, exhaustion, and numbness in his hands were classic indicators of the disease. Larry's job depended on manual dexterity, so he became forced to take medical leave. We had experienced good results using bee venom injections in several patients with MS, so Larry thought we might be able to help him. We did a full medical work-up, but the results were inconclusive.

We proceeded with a series of toxicity tests, looking for factors that might have led to the onset of his symptoms (see chapter 7 for more details on toxicity tests). We found that Larry had abnormally high levels of lead in his body. We then reviewed his medical history and found that he had reported classic symptoms of lead poisoning: abdominal and bone pain. Lead is also known to cause neurological problems that can mimic those of MS. We concluded that Larry had been given the wrong diagnosis: He was actually suffering from lead toxicity.

might be done to confirm the diagnosis, and a treatment program follows. The name of the problem usually describes the type of damage that the disease has wrought or the part of the body that's affected. The treatment is based on a model called the "standard of care," which means that the physician treats the disease, not the person, using the standard textbook approach. This model is not designed to factor in the biochemical individuality of each patient and the uniqueness of his or her situation.

This method of health care delivery works very well in certain cases, especially when a patient's problem and the doctor's diagnosis are a perfect fit. However, in many cases, the fit is not quite so perfect. When a doctor can't identify a clear-cut cause, he or she treats the symptoms alone, often with medications to suppress them, and the patient never really gets better. Temporarily stopping the pain with a drug or cutting out the tissue that is diseased, only to have the problem show up somewhere else, is not the same as treating the source of the problem. In some cases, the source of the problem is separate from the site of the disease.

For example, arthritis means inflammation in the joint, and gastritis means inflammation in the stomach. These names are descriptive only—they tell us nothing about why the inflammation has occurred. However, from the point of view of naturopathic medicine, these states of tissue inflammation arise from disorders in other parts of the body. A person with arthritis could actually have a digestive problem, and gastric inflammation could be the result of extreme anxiety and stress. In natural healing, the reason for an illness is more important than its name. The cure begins with the cause.

And toxins are often the real source of the problem. Toxicity syndromes (disorders characterized by a host of symptoms due to toxic reactions to certain substances) are the result of exposure to these toxins, which poison the blood. Such substances may be created inside the body or come from outside. In either case, if the body can't get rid of them, they become harmful. Medical practitioners of the East have understood the concept of "poisoned blood" for thousands of years, but until recently, no scientific tests could confirm the presence of toxins in the body, identify them precisely, and accurately measure levels of contamination. Today, new tests (like the one for intestinal permeability, which confirms that toxins from bacterial by-products in the intestines can leak into the bloodstream) are increasing our ability to diagnose and treat toxicity syndromes.

Toxic Synergism

Synergy describes the combined effect of different actions or parts on a whole system, and it's an important concept to understand when we look at how toxins affect health. The synergistic action of toxins means that the consequences of one compound acting on the organism (for example, the lead found in food and water), when combined with the consequences of another compound (for example, mercury released from dental amalgams), will cause more damage to cells than the simple sum of the two.

Each person has a built-in capacity to adapt to a variety of metabolic stressors and cope with the demands they put on the body. But there are limits to our biological tolerance. Exposure to the multiple toxins found in medications, food, water, and air pushes the human adaptive mechanism beyond its limits. Amid this barrage of toxins the body can no longer protect itself. As a consequence, people are suffering from a problem called toxic synergy. It is creating new problems for which the traditional Western medical model has no standard of care.

In natural healing, the reason for an illness is more important than its name. The cure begins with the cause.

An example of toxic synergism can be seen in chemicals that can mimic estrogen activity. Compounds found in plastics, such as bisphenol A, are released into food and water

Gulf War Syndrome: A Case of Toxic Synergy?

Of the 750,000 persons involved in the Gulf War, about 100,000 have complained of neurological symptoms of unknown cause. Although no single cause has been clearly implicated, one contributing factor might be the simultaneous exposure to multiple chemical agents. To protect their health, service personnel were exposed to the anti-nerve gas agent pyristigmine bromide, the insect repellent DEET, and the insecticide permethrin.

In a study using hens, exposure to each of these compounds individually resulted in minimal levels of neurotoxicity. However, the combination of two agents at the same doses produced higher levels of neurotoxicity, and the combination of all three agents resulted in even higher levels of toxicity. The Gulf War has shown us that combinations of toxic substances can have unpredictable results.

when exposed to heat. Such compounds have the ability to bind to estrogen receptors in the cells. The cells respond as if estrogen is actually present when, in fact, it is not. When other compounds that are known to mimic estrogen, such as those found in pesticides, are added to one another, the effect is greatly magnified. This disrupts the normal hormonal balance in both men and women and increases the risk for cancer.

Toxins are damaging the ecology of the environment both inside and outside our bodies. Compounds that have never before been encountered are poisoning the cellular machinery and disturbing genetic transcription (the way the information carried in our DNA translates into cellular function). Humans have always had to adapt to destructive forces in nature and naturally occurring poisons, but never to so many new compounds and forces at one time. These conditions demand an unprecedented adaptive response from our bodies.

Toxic Ecology

Most of the ecological nightmares predicted by Rachel Carson in her book *The Silent Spring* have come to pass. As a result of pollution, certain species of animal and plant life have disappeared. Pesticides, designed to kill biological organisms, are part of our food chain. Cancer is increasingly prevalent—Carson herself died of breast cancer.

What she didn't predict was the multitude of compounds now flooding our environment that act in lethal synergy with one another. This toxic synergy was not recognized until recently. According to current studies, forty carcinogens may be in our drinking water. Sixty carcinogens are released into the air by industrial processes, and another sixty-six are sprayed on food crops as pesticides. Unfortunately, no definitive research has evaluated the effect of all such chemicals in our diet and drinking water acting at the same time.

Manufacturers of industrial chemicals are not accountable to the same safety laws that govern the pharmaceutical industry when it comes to introducing foreign compounds for human use. According to the rules that control the chemical industry, the public bears the burden of proving that these substances are harmful. Chemical manufacturers are not obliged to prove that their products are safe. Although most countries now recognize the terrible effect of the toxic environment on human health, no real solutions have been offered. The U.S. Environmental Protection Agency has released some staggering statistics about how many millions of pounds of toxic chemicals have been released into the environment through 1994 (see table 2.2).

Table 2.2. *Amount of Toxic Chemicals Released into the Environment Through 1994*

Location	Amount
On-site land	4 million pounds (2.5 million pounds in 1992)
Surface water	25 million pounds
Air	42 million pounds
On-site deep-well injection	40 million pounds
Total reported release	111 million pounds
Total estimated release	2.2 billion pounds

Toxicity Syndromes

Many health problems have been definitively linked in a cause-and-effect relationship with exposure to specific toxins, including those that we willingly expose ourselves to by our lifestyle choices. Keep in mind that foods, even those normally considered good for you, can be considered toxins for those individuals who are sensitive to them. Table 2.3 charts the relationship between these factors and some common health problems and diseases. Sometimes the health problems and disease names that doctors give in relation to their patients hide or ignore the underlying cause of cell dysfunction, which might be a toxicity syndrome.

Signs of Toxicity

Toxicity syndromes are common but often go undetected. Liver disorders, frequent drug reactions, a sensitivity to synthetic fragrances (such as those in air fresheners, shampoos, and laundry detergents), frequent edema or swelling (especially around the eyes), and a feeling of being hungover without having consumed alcohol are all indicators that you may have a toxicity-related problem. Table 2.4 outlines some of the symptoms that you should take as warning signs of toxicity.

Many health problems have been definitively linked with exposure to specific toxins, including those that we expose ourselves to by our lifestyle choices.

Some of your body's systems are particularly vulnerable to certain toxins. Figure 2.2 illustrates the possible dangers to which you might be exposed. The sections that follow describe in detail some conditions that should serve as red flags to indicate possible toxicity. You can also use the questionnaire at the back of the book to get your own numerical "score" for each type of toxic exposure. Your total score gives you some idea of just how toxic your body may be.

Tooth and Gum Diseases

Pay special attention to your teeth and gums. The condition of the mouth is pivotal. Untreated cavities, gum disease,

How do you know whether you are at risk and need to be evaluated for toxicity syndromes? Look for the signs of toxicity, which can manifest as either generally poor health, with symptoms that include headaches, arthritic-type pain, lethargy, overweight, low resistance to bacterial and viral infections, or as one of the following diseases:

Cancer. It is well known that high levels of exposure to carcinogens, coupled with altered detoxification enzymes responsible for their breakdown, significantly increase one's susceptibility to cancer. Alcohol, cigarettes, medications, and pollutants have an altering effect on these enzymes. For example, bladder cancer is linked to exposure to industrial chemicals, breast cancer is linked to pesticides, and lung cancer is linked to smoking.

Autoimmune disease. Some toxins, such as altered bowel flora, pesticides, and mercury, undermine the immune system and so are associated with the onset and progression of autoimmune diseases such as lupus and rheumatoid arthritis.

bacteria-filled root canals, silver fillings, tooth implants, and nickel crowns can be the primary source of toxicity that affects the entire body. Poor oral hygiene may be the cause of gum disease or tooth decay, but these conditions could also indicate that the diet includes too many damaging foods and insufficient nutrients.

Information about oral toxicity has been available since 1928. Weston Price, a dentist, studied the effects of chronic dental infections on overall health. In his paper "Dental Infections, Their Dangers and Prevention," Price described how

Neurological disease. Exposure to pesticides, metals, mercury, and other toxins, and the biochemical defects they trigger significantly affect the nervous system and negatively impact brain function. The situation is even more critical when there is an inadequate intake of essential nutrients, especially antioxidants—the dietary factors that protect the body from oxidative damage caused by the unstable, reactive oxygen molecules, known as free radicals, normally circulating in the body.

Arthritis. Arthritis pain may be related to a toxic reaction to specific foods (food allergies), dehydration from inadequate intake of water (a very common problem) and bowel toxemia.

Bowel disease. This condition can be the result of food allergies or an imbalance of normal bowel flora.

Immune diseases. These disorders are related to pesticides, industrial chemicals (dioxins), and mercury in the blood, and the presence of harmful bacteria in the bowel.

Cardiovascular disease. This problem has been linked to the presence of heavy metals in the bloodstream.

teeth harboring anaerobic bacteria, especially in cases in which root canal work has been done, could injure the health of genetically susceptible individuals. Price's work has never been followed up by other researchers, but many patients, doctors, and dentists have observed the accuracy of his findings. In our clinic, we have had several cases of facial neuralgia—extreme pain in the sensory and motor nerves of the face—that were relieved after the removal of root canal teeth and cavitation.

Oral diseases, especially those caused by toxic reactions, can have serious consequences. It's important for

Table 2.3. *Common Health Problems and Their Toxic Triggers*

Disease	Trigger
Alzheimer's Disease	
Metals	Aluminum, lead
Chemicals	Pesticides
Allergies	
Chemicals	Formaldehyde
Foods	Wheat, dairy products, yeast, and any other foods that cause negative reactions
Lifestyle habits	Smoking
Anemia	
Metals	Lead poisoning
Foods	Any foods that cause negative reactions, nutrient deficiencies
Lifestyle habits	Alcohol
Angina	
Metals	Lead
Foods	Any foods that cause allergic reactions
	Overconsumption of sugar and unhealthy fats
Arthritis	
Foods	Coffee, chocolate, any foods that cause allergic reactions
Lifestyle habits	Smoking
Asthma	
Metals	Lead
Chemicals	Reaction to chemical odors and air pollution
Foods	Milk products, any foods that cause allergic reactions
Lifestyle habits	Mildew in building ventilation

Table 2.3. *Common Health Problems and Their Toxic Triggers (continued)*

Disease	Trigger
Autoimmune Disease	
Metals	Mercury
Chemicals	Silicone breast implants
Foods	Nutritional deficiencies
Behavior Disorders	
Foods	Food intolerance, sugar intolerance, sensitivity to food dyes
Colitis	
Foods	Any foods that cause allergic reactions
Cancer	
Chemicals	Pesticides, radiation, low-frequency electromagnetic fields
Foods	Overconsumption of meats cooked on a charcoal fire
Lifestyle habits	Smoking, alcohol
Cataracts	
Chemicals	Industrial pollutants, steroids
Foods	Antioxidant-deficient diet
Lifestyle habits	Smoking
Colic	
Metals	Lead
Foods	Any foods that cause negative reactions
Coronary Artery Disease	
Metals	Lead, cadmium
Chemicals	Air pollution
Foods	Alcohol, fried foods, excessive consumption of meat, sugar, and refined flour
Lifestyle habits	Smoking

Table 2.3. *Common Health Problems and Their Toxic Triggers (continued)*

Disease	Trigger
Diabetes	
Foods	Allergic reactions to dairy products, gluten sensitivity
Chronic Fatigue Syndrome	
Metals	Lead, mercury
Chemicals	Pesticides
Foods	Any foods that cause negative reactions
Lifestyle habits	Overwork, persistent worry
Infertility	
Metals	Mercury
Chemicals	Pesticides
Fibromyalgia	
Chemicals	Pesticides
Fractures	
Chemicals	Fluoride (causes "brittle bone syndrome")
Headaches	
Metals	Mercury
Foods	Any foods that cause negative reactions
High Cholesterol	
Metals	Cadmium, lead
Foods	Caffeine, fried foods
Lifestyle habits	Alcohol
Hypertension	
Metals	Lead, cadmium, mercury
Kidney Disease	
Metals	Mercury
Foods	Any foods that cause negative reactions

Table 2.3. *Common Health Problems and Their Toxic Triggers (continued)*

Disease	Trigger
Liver Disorders	
Lifestyle habits	Alcohol
Macular Degeneration (impaired vision due to deterioration of the central portion of the retina)	
Lifestyle habits	Smoking
Multiple Sclerosis	
Metals	Mercury
Chemicals	Industrial pollutants
Foods	Any foods that cause allergic reactions
Parkinson's Disease	
Chemicals	Pesticides
Lifestyle habits	Smoking

Table 2.4. *Symptoms of Toxicity by Body System*

Body System	Symptoms
Central Nervous System	Cognitive problems, poor memory, numbness in the extremities
Immune System	Frequent colds, night sweats, sudden onset of allergies
Gastrointestinal System	Bloating, pain, diarrhea, belching, unpleasant smelling gas
Musculoskeletal System	Paresthesia (numbness or tingling), pain, weakness, fatigue
Sensory	Vertigo, extreme sensitivity to odors
Skin	Hives, eczema, itching

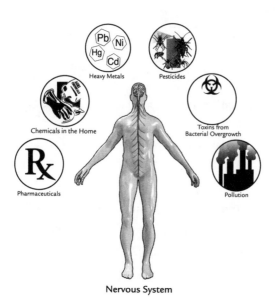

Nervous System

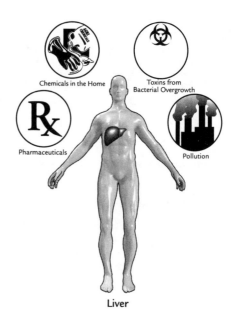

Liver

Figure 2.2

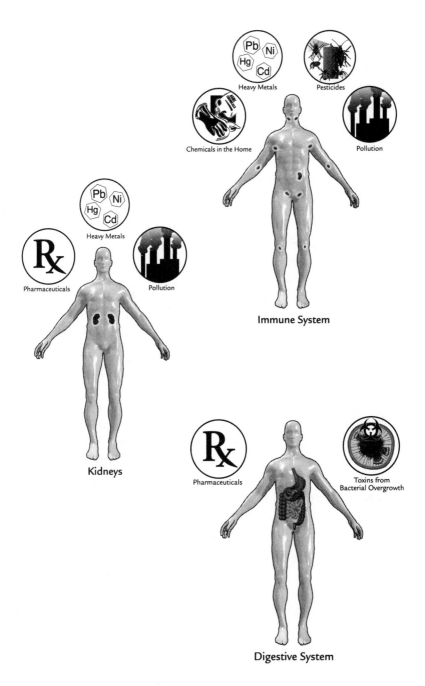

Figure 2.2 (continued)

patients who have a history of chronic health complaints to have a thorough dental review to ensure that infections, cavitation, metals, and galvanic currents (electrical currents produced by the chemical reactions of metals in the mouth) are not causing disorders in the highly sensitive area of the oral cavity. Our experience has shown that this is one of the most important areas to investigate when pursuing the cause of chronic illness. The dental examination should be done by a qualified practitioner of what is called biological dentistry. (See appendix for information about how to locate a biological dentist.)

Fibromyalgia and Chronic Fatigue Syndrome

A recent study showed that patients with diagnoses of chronic fatigue syndrome, fibromyalgia, and multiple chemical sensitivity syndrome could not be distinguished on the basis of symptoms. The study indicates that these are not separate diseases but different forms of the same illness. These poorly differentiated disorders are probably caused by many environmental factors.

Several studies indicate that chemical toxicity and immune-system breakdown provoke the disorders. At our clinic, many patients ask whether a treatment exists for fibromyalgia and chronic fatigue syndrome. Detoxification therapy has been shown to be effective and stands out as one of the only coherent approaches to healing people with these debilitating health problems. We are convinced that these mysterious disorders are indications that the stress of environmental toxins is more than some people can handle.

Nervous System Disorders

The central nervous system is extremely sensitive to toxins in the bloodstream, and brain activity depends on a delicate electrochemical balance of hormones, neurotransmitters, and brain peptides. Toxins can disturb this natural balance, and the results can range from a sense of persistent mental "fog" (cognitive impairment) to serious diseases such as Alzheimer's, Parkinson's, and motor neuron disease.

For example, polychloride biphenyls, better known as PCBs, are a class of common industrial compounds known to be carcinogenic and neurotoxic. In 1979, 2,000 people were poisoned in Taiwan from cooking with oil contaminated with PCBs. Symptoms in 44 percent of the victims were mainly neurological, sensory, and motor nerve conduction, leading some researchers to conclude that protecting brain cells from these toxins can prevent brain aging and neurodegenerative diseases. The central nervous system is also highly vulnerable to damage from free radicals, the "chaotic" oxygen molecules that scavenge electrons from other cells and cause oxidative damage.

If you have any doubt that circulating toxins can create altered brain states, you need only recall your mental condition "the morning after," when alcohol consumption has left you with a hangover. In fact, people with an overburdened and sluggish detoxification system often feel as if they have a hangover (but without the headache) all the time. People who are exposed to toxins such as pesticides report this type of distorted awareness. Depending on the type of poison, the debilitating effects can last for years.

Almost everyone who undergoes detoxification experiences razor-sharp mental clarity by the end of the process. The message here is that the nervous system is highly sensitive to toxins in the blood.

Parkinson's Disease   Evidence suggests that environmental toxins influence the onset of Parkinson's disease. The disease is not viral in origin and is not an autoimmune disorder. We now know that Parkinson's disease is found more frequently in industrialized countries. The exact cause or causes are still unknown, but some researchers suspect that they relate to heavy metals, chemicals, pesticides, fertilizers used in farming, contaminated well water, and wood pulp manufacturing. It's very common for Parkinson's patients to have been exposed to pesticides and petroleum derivatives.

Parkinson's may also be the result of an inherited vulnerability to toxins caused by poor detoxification abilities. Biochemical lab testing shows that there are decreased concentrations of antioxidants in the brain cells of Parkinson's patients, which suggests that the damage could be caused by free radicals.

Alzheimer's Disease   Alzheimer's is a disease whose main symptom is brain damage, which likely results from a variety of toxins in the environment. It is especially difficult to treat because, as illustrated by the pyramid of priorities described in chapter 1, toxins have penetrated to the very core of the organism.

The disease has been related to an inherited detoxification weakness and to toxicity caused by exposure to aluminum, mercury, pesticides, and wheat gluten (to which many people have an undiagnosed allergy). Several studies showed that the brain tissue of Alzheimer's patients had high levels of mercury. Pesticides, which are powerful inhibitors of neurotransmitters and cause paralysis of nerve transmission, have also been implicated. These chemicals can induce symptoms that are very similar to those of Alzheimer's and might be related to its cause. One doctor has reported that many of his Alzheimer's patients are sensitive to wheat gliadin/gluten.

Multiple Chemical Sensitivity Syndrome

Exposure to the huge number of chemicals present in most people's everyday lives can cause a wide range of immune and neurological diseases. Our food supply alone bombards the body with a profusion of toxins. What we eat contains pesticides, bleaching agents, preservatives, artificial coloring, waxes, fumigants, hormones, and antibiotics. Fast foods might be fried in rancid oils and fats that have been rendered unhealthy by overheating, nuts and grains are often contaminated with molds, and carcinogens are found in meats cooked over charcoal. Those who suffer from multiple chemical sensitivity (MCS) often go from one specialist to another trying to get help, until someone recognizes that these patients are exhibiting reactions to a variety of different chemical compounds that often produce symptoms in more than one organ system. Such a condition is hard to diagnose, and it is generally not even acknowledged as a disease entity by those who practice mainstream medicine. But MCS is real, and it is treatable with detoxification therapy.

Signs of Health

You can measure your health status in ways other than blood pressure readings, stress tests, or laboratory analysis of blood. You can take stock of your well-being every day. Take a close look in the mirror and study your reflection. In our clinic, we can see whether patients are suffering from toxicity as soon as we look at their faces. Ask yourself some simple questions about your mood, your body functions, and your ability to get through your day and enjoy your life. You can personally review your body's systems and parts for signs of toxic stress. Give yourself a daily checkup using the following guidelines. If you answer yes to the questions, you may be suffering from toxicity.

Mind, Emotions, and Attitude

The mind and the emotions are two good indicators of overall health. An inability to think clearly and focus attention, volatile moods and depression, or a lack of enthusiasm or positive interest in your life can be clues that you're suffering from a toxic overload.

How are you functioning mentally?

- Do you have difficulty concentrating?
- Do you feel mentally sluggish?
- Does your thinking seem slow or fuzzy?

How are you functioning emotionally?

- Do you have a generally negative outlook?
- Do you experience sudden, uncontrollable mood swings?
- Do you feel apathetic, dull, or listless?

Energy Level

The human organism was designed to work hard for a full eighty years of life. Healthy people of all ages have enough energy to labor all day and then "play" at night. Energy comes from proper cellular metabolism, a correct balance of hormones, and maintaining precise biochemical equilibrium in the nervous system. Energy is also intimately linked to our emotional state: Attitudes affect energy levels and vice versa. For example, depressed people often sleep much more than normal, and sick people tend to feel "blue." Not having the energy you once had or feeling that you don't have enough time to do all the things you want and need to do in life could indicate something about the level of toxins in your body.

How's your energy level?

- Do you experience extreme and persistent fatigue?
- Do you feel lethargic most of the time?
- Does ordinary activity leave you exhausted?
- Are you tired, even after a good night's sleep?

Skin

The skin is the largest of our organs and has multiple responsibilities. It provides a protective barrier, helps maintain normal body temperature, and is a medium for the elimination of toxins. Healthy skin is elastic and young looking, with a vibrancy that comes from within. Toxicity and sickness leave skin dry, tired and old looking, blemished, or spotty with uneven color (especially noticeable on the face). It loses its normal texture and appears loose and sagging. You can usually spot a smoker because of the dusky appearance of his or her skin.

Detoxification therapy has been shown to be effective and stands out as one of the only coherent approaches to healing chronic disease.

The coloring of the skin of the face can be a good indication of fatigue, poor nutrition, liver disease, anemia, and chronic disease. A ruddy complexion indicates that blood is circulating well through the digestive tract. Such a complexion comes from fresh air, regular exercise, proper digestion, and adequate rest. A red nose indicates inflammation in the stomach or liver. An extremely pale complexion indicates weakness of circulation. A yellow or slightly green complexion indicates anemia or poor liver function.

Internal imbalances also manifest themselves in how your body smells. A strong, unpleasant odor indicates fermentation and putrefaction in the intestines. Disease and sickness have a distinctive odor, one that you can smell whenever you walk into a hospital. As patients become detoxified, they emanate a "cleaner" smell through their skin.

How's your skin?

• Is your skin dull colored, pale, grayish, or slightly yellow?

• Does your skin seem loose, flabby?

• Does your skin give off a sharp, sour, unpleasant odor?

• Is your complexion unusually pale or sallow?

• Is your face marred by blemishes?

• Do you have poor facial skin tone with much wrinkling and sagging?

Tongue

The tongue is an accurate diagnostic tool, but conventional medical doctors generally don't use it to evaluate organ function. Tongue diagnosis is used extensively and effectively in the traditional medical systems of India and China, as well as by homeopathic physicians.

The tongue should have a healthy pink color, with a slight coating that is milky but transparent. Indications that the liver or digestive organs are not functioning properly include a tongue that appears swollen, as evidenced by teeth marks on either side; is thin and dry with a shrunken or flattened appearance; has a yellow, grayish-white, or thick coating; or is shiny without any coating at all.

The condition of your tongue can give you information about your intestinal tract. To examine your tongue, finish your last meal of the day by 5 P.M. and be sure that meal does not include any meat. The next morning, look at your tongue in the mirror right after you wake up, before you've had breakfast, had a drink of water, or even brushed your teeth. A coated tongue indicates weak digestion; the thicker the coating, the more serious the need for detoxification therapy.

How's your tongue's appearance?

• Is it swollen?

• Does it appear shrunken or flattened?

• Is it coated with a yellow, grayish-white, or thick film?

• Is your tongue shiny?

Eyes

The eyes are correctly called the "windows of the soul," and they also offer a view of the state of your health. In a happy, healthy individual, the eyes appear bright and lustrous. The whites of the eyes are clear. There is no discoloration or swelling around the eyes. Dark circles around the eyes, bags, or swelling are signs of a disturbance in either kidney or liver function. However, the relationship between dark circles around the eyes and problems with kidney or liver function is not accepted in Western medicine and shouldn't be used as the only basis of determining the severity of organ dysfunction.

How's the appearance of your eyes?

• Do you have dark circles around your eyes?

• Are your eyelids swollen?

• Are your eyelids inflamed?

• Are there bags under your eyes?

• Are your eyes bloodshot?

• Is there yellow in the whites of your eyes?

Digestion

When your body has to absorb the toxic chemistry of bowel fermentation, pathogenic bacteria, and toxic substances called amines (ammonia derivatives) from the putrefaction and fermentation of protein in the intestinal tract, you feel ill. Headaches, tired eyes, low energy, lack of hunger and thirst, constipation, abdominal fullness, and mental dullness are classic symptoms of the presence of these digestive tract toxins. Also, belching, bloating, gas, abdominal pain, and heartburn after eating are indications of some sort of bowel inflammation or infection. Eating should be a painless event and result in none of these symptoms. You should feel energetic and have a satisfied feeling of well-being after your meals.

How's your digestion?

- Do you frequently suffer from heartburn or indigestion?

- Do you experience bloating after eating?

- Do you have excessive gas?

- Do you experience abdominal discomfort after eating?

- Do certain foods aggravate your stomach?

Bowels

The quality of the stool tells you about how well you're digesting the food you eat. If you have enough fiber in your diet, your stool is soft but formed, and you have a bowel movement regularly, that is, once or twice every day. A loose, unformed stool indicates intestinal irritation. A greasy stool that floats often means that fats are not being properly broken down and that pancreas or gallbladder function is poor. Offensive odor indicates intestinal putrefaction and fermentation. A bowel movement should be a healthy discharge of food waste, not a path for the removal of environmental and self-generated toxins.

How are your bowels?

- Do you have fewer than one bowel movement a day?

- Are your stools loose and unformed?

- Do your stools contain undigested bits of food?

- Are your bowel movements uncomfortable? Do you have to strain?

- Do your stools float?

- Do your bowel movements have a strong, offensive odor?

- Is there any rectal pain or bleeding?

- Is there mucus in your stool?

Urine

You should produce 500 to 2,500 milliliters (or 1 to 5 quarts) of urine a day. You should also empty your bladder every time you drink something. Urine should be light, with a slight color and almost no odor. Certain nutritional supplements such as vitamin C or riboflavin will typically turn your urine bright yellow. Dehydration and toxicity syndromes cause urine to be dark yellow in color with a frothy or oily appearance.

How's your urine?

- Does your urine have an offensive odor?

- Is it dark yellow in color?

- Is it frothy?

- Do you urinate infrequently?

Joints

Flexibility and ease of movement depends on healthy joints. Joints have special nutritional needs, and a clear relationship exists between the digestive tract and your joints. The intestinal tract can leak material into the bloodstream that causes inflammation in the joints. Many patients with food allergies report that their arthritis gets worse if they eat food that irritates their intestinal system.

Toxins in the bloodstream can damage delicate joint tissue, resulting in joint pain either throughout the musculoskeletal system or in isolated regions. Slight swelling or aching joints in the morning could be caused by toxins, and degenerative arthritis or a worsening of arthritic symptoms should alert you to the possibility of toxic stress.

How are your joints?

- Are your joints sore after waking?

- Do you experience pain in joints after slight exertion?

- Do you experience pain in joints after eating certain foods?

Abdominal Muscle Tone

The abdomen should have good muscle tone without any protrusion or swelling. Chronic bloating alters the natural tone of the abdomen. As intestinal health breaks down, digestive organs can slip out of place (prolapse). This shifting of the position of intestinal structures means that they don't function properly. Intestinal toxicity can also lead to irritation of the muscles of the back and pelvis, weakening them and causing poor posture.

How's your posture?

- Does your abdomen tend to hang out?

- Does the surface of your abdomen appear unevenly and irregularly distended?

- If you have a protruding belly, do you experience lower back pain?

Nails

The nails of the fingers and toes should be rigid without any discoloration or topographical changes. Any changes in the normal appearance of the nails can indicate any one of the following: mineral deficiencies, nutritional imbalances, and improper liver function.

How are your nails?

- Are they ridged?

- Are they split?

- Are they spotted?

- Are they crumbling?

Your answers to all the questions we've posed are useful tools for a do-it-yourself assessment of your physical, emotional, and mental health. They can serve as a toxic yardstick—a quick, easy way to measure just how much toxic exposure is costing you. But toxins are doing their damage long before you may be able to see and feel their effects. They attack the body at the most fundamental level, altering cellular function and polluting the fluids in which cells are bathed. So, in the next chapter, we explain what cells do, how they do it, and why it's so important that the "sea" of blood and lymph in which they "swim" is clean and free flowing.

CHAPTER 3

Cells, Blood, and Lymph

- **The Cell: The Basic Unit of Life**
- **Blood: Aqua Vita, or the Water of Life**
- **Lymph: The Other Vital Fluid**

When considering the health of the body, we generally focus on external parts, internal organs, and systemic functions. However, the fundamental building blocks of these parts, organs, and functions are cells, the spaces around those cells, and the fluid environment that surrounds them. Understanding how your body works, what makes you sick, and what keeps you healthy entails understanding cell structure and activity. Cells are the basic unit of life; blood brings them nourishment, and lymphatic fluid carries waste products away. The three modules of our program have been designed to address the needs of these basic body components.

The Cell: The Basic Unit of Life

Every single cell in the body consists of a nucleus, mitochondria, and a cell membrane (see figure 3.1). These three key structures form the basis of the metabolic activity that keeps us alive. The nucleus contains DNA, the body's biochemical memory and control center. Mitochondria produce specialized molecules to make energy. Membranes are the medium through which cells communicate with each other.

The Nucleus

The nucleus is the only structure in the cell that has "memory," and it uses this "knowledge," chemically encoded in its DNA, to direct all the activities of the cell. DNA contains a library of instructions that govern every bodily function. The nucleus knows many biochemical languages that it can translate for all the parts of the cell and all the parts of the body. It sends and receives cellular messages that travel through the bloodstream. These messages tell cells to manufacture different types of proteins that regulate their activity.

How Toxins Damage DNA Exposure to toxins, notably industrial chemicals known to be cancer-causing agents, disrupts activity in the nucleus by damaging DNA. Toxins damage DNA in two ways. Some toxins have the ability to alter and confuse the expression of DNA, as in the estrogen-mimicking effect of pesticides. Second, as toxins are broken down, free radicals are created that steal electrons from DNA, thereby changing its chemical code (see figure 3.2). Carcinogens, like benzopyrene from cigarette smoke, create dangerous free radicals, which attack the DNA of the liver,

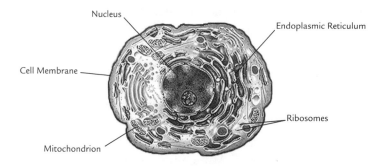

Nucleus

Endoplasmic Reticulum

Cell Membrane

Ribosomes

Mitochondrion

Diagram of a Cell

Figure 3.1

The three key structures of a cell are the nucleus,
the mitochondria, and the cell membrane.

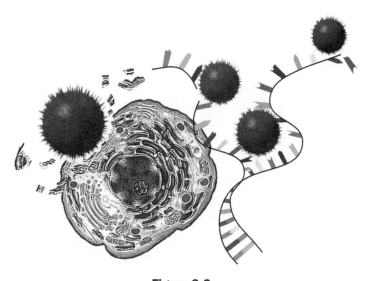

Figure 3.2

Free radicals damage cellular structures and disrupt DNA.

arteries, and central nervous system. Once the memory encoded in the DNA has been upset, no drugs or treatments
can repair it. Although detoxification therapy cannot undo
the harm done to DNA by exposure to chemicals, radiation,

and other toxins, it can strengthen the body's own repair mechanisms and provide protection against further harm.

Mitochondria

The mitochondria are the power-generating plants of the cell. They turn oxygen and glucose (sugar) into energy and make it available to fuel muscles and organs. The mitochondria are always at work. Mitochondria use oxygen and glucose to make ATP (adenosine triphosphate), the substance that drives all the chemical reactions inside the cell. If the production of ATP stops, all the cell's activities grind to a halt. Our need for oxygen is an expression of the relentless demands of the mitochondria. If the supply of oxygen to the mitochondria is interrupted, it is life threatening. Neurons in the brain begin to die within three minutes of not having oxygen because of the high energy needs of these specialized cells. Other key cells in vital tissues soon follow.

However, oxygen can also be dangerous. As it goes about its work of generating energy inside of the mitochondria, oxygen produces free radicals that damage vital cellular components and disrupt the delicate process of making ATP. Our bodies need a steady supply of antioxidant nutrients to protect cells from the assaults of free radicals.

How Toxins Damage Mitochondria   Free radicals are also produced when toxins work their way into the mitochondria. Unlike other parts of the cell, mitochondria lack detoxification enzymes that can break down toxic chemicals and heavy metals. Detoxification therapy helps prevent the formation of these dangerous free radicals by enhancing the breakdown of toxins in the liver so that they are eliminated before they invade the mitochondria.

During exercise, the mitochondria create organic acids (metabolic by-products, also known as acids of metabolism). The blood is supposed to carry these waste products away, taking them to the liver and kidneys for eventual dismantling and elimination. If it does not, these acids become damaging toxins. People who cannot detoxify their cells of waste products from mitochondria tend to get sick.

Although detoxification therapy cannot undo the harm done to DNA by exposure to chemicals, radiation, and other toxins, it can strengthen the body's own repair mechanisms and provide protection against further harm.

Research by Dr. D. I. Arnold at Oxford University showed that the cells of a patient sick with myalgia encephalomyelitis (ME), another name for chronic fatigue syndrome and fibromyalgia, were not able to get rid of waste acids after only moderate exercise. Our program outlined in chapter 8 will help you improve your body's ability to deal with these waste acids.

The Cell Membrane

The cell membrane, a fuzzy film of fat that surrounds the cell, is almost as important as the cell itself. It serves as a kind of communications center, containing millions of tiny antennae, receptors, and entryways that control what passes in and out of the cell body. A sort of listening-and-receiving device, the cell membrane also displays "address" codes used by the immune system. These codes are chemical markers that help the immune system differentiate between the body's own cells and foreign invaders, such as viruses and bacteria.

Neurotransmitters, brain peptides, hormones, and endorphins generate their own unique "messages" that bind to cell membrane receptors. The nervous, endocrine, and immune systems must constantly communicate with each other.

Many practitioners of alternative medicine realize that the basis of their efforts is to create a healthy extracellular matrix.

When the cell membrane is not properly formed, the intercellular communications network shuts down. Cells can't make contact with one another, are unable to receive and transmit their messages, and thus are cut off from the rest of the body. There is a breakdown in the unified knowledge of the cell, which no longer "understands" how it is connected to other cells.

How Toxins Deform the Cell Membrane   When the cell loses the ability to detoxify itself, toxic chemicals bind to cell membrane receptors, producing what we call "toxic noise." Like static on the radio, this "noise" interferes with cell-to-cell communication, impairing the brain's ability to function normally and upsetting communication in the immune, nervous, and endocrine systems. Many toxins, especially heavy metals and fat-soluble pesticides, have an affinity for the fat and protein structures of cell membranes.

Heavy metals, such as mercury, bind with the sulfhydryl protein embedded in the cell membrane and alter the address code. Certain white blood cells, called natural killer (NK) cells, are the Secret Service agents of the immune system. If a cell membrane does not display the correct address code, NK cells treat it as a foreign invader, and their job is to destroy it. Autoimmune diseases, in which the immune system attacks the body's own cells, are an outcome of this alteration. A toxin such as mercury is known to easily induce autoimmune disease in the kidneys of animals. We believe that it can also generate autoimmune disease in humans.

The primary aim of detoxification therapy is to clean the blood. We've found that changing and optimizing the diet and stimulating circulation encourage the organs of the immune system to filter the blood.

For the cell surface markers to express the correct address codes, the cell membrane must be soft, not stiff. The softer the membranes, the more resilient and accommodating they are to communication and transport. The type of fats used to build membranes determines how pliable they

The Benefits of Essential Fatty Acids

Cultures, like the Eskimo, that eat a diet high in these essential fats have a very low incidence of autoimmune disease, whereas essential fatty acid deficiencies appear to predispose people to a wide variety of immune system disorders and inflammatory diseases. It's interesting to note that essential fatty acids are known mainly for treating diseases of the immune system, such as asthma, arthritis, and cancer. These diseases are associated with inflammation, poor cell recognition, and membrane damage, all of which are disorders related to the cell membrane and hallmarks of pesticide and heavy-metal poisoning.

A group of researchers in Australia found a pattern of abnormally shaped red blood cells in the blood of patients suffering from chronic fatigue and chemical exposure. Their findings suggested that chemicals had interfered with the membrane structure of red blood cells. These cells were inflexible and had difficulty sliding through the small capillary spaces to deliver oxygen. This meant that these sites were starved for oxygen. Common chemicals that pollute our environment have a high affinity for the fatty cell membranes, and it is possible that these poisons were incorporated into the cell membrane and altered its structure. Poor dietary fatty acid intake leads to membranes that are more easily damaged by toxins.

will be. The wrong kind of fats—such as those from a diet high in deep-fried foods, rancid oils, and margarine—leave the membranes brittle and weak. Essential fatty acids—found

Johanna Budwig, a leading authority on essential fatty acids, especially flax oil, noted in experiments that the animals who had proper fatty acids were able to withstand the cancer-causing effects of benzopyrenes in cigarette smoke. She noted that the electron-rich nutrition of flax oil is capable of counteracting harmful influences.

Attention deficit disorder (ADD) might also be linked to damaged cell membranes. Because cells with damaged membranes are highly susceptible to confusion from "toxic noise," they misinterpret biochemical signals and send out incorrect messages. We believe that this is an excellent model to explain the problems found in children with ADD. It's possible that in these children brain cell membranes have been damaged as a result of too much of the wrong type of fat in combination with environmental toxins such as lead, which has been linked to learning disorders. A dietary shortage of essential fatty acids can also lead to nerve damage, and there is strong evidence that fats have a significant effect on the binding of chemical transmitters in the brain, which affects mood and behavior.

Children with ADD have also been found to be deficient in DHA (decohexanoic acid, a fatty acid critical for healthy brain cell membranes). DHA could provide a safe alternative to the drug Ritalin, and further research on treating ADD should focus on cell membrane nutrition. For a thorough discussion of fats and brain health, see Michael Schmidt's book *Smart Fats* (Berkeley, CA: Frog Ltd., 1977).

in such foods as cold-water seafood and oils made from flaxseed, borage, sunflower seeds, sesame seeds, and walnuts, and in the supplement evening primrose oil—provide the nutrients needed to maintain flexible, smooth cell membranes. Such healthy membranes provide a better, clearer set of address codes for the immune system. Many doctors who practice detoxification medicine stress the need to supplement toxin-exposed patients with flax oil and borage oil, two types of essential fatty acids, in order to repair damage done to cell membranes.

Essential fatty acids create healthy membranes that support both immune and detoxification activity. Two tablespoons of flaxseed oil daily is the recommended dose for healthy cell membranes and maximum protection against toxins. An excellent overview of the therapeutic uses of essential fatty acids is found in Udo Erasmus's book, *The Complete Guide to Fats and Oils in Health and Nutrition* (Vancouver: Alive Books, 1986).

The Extracellular Matrix: The Cell's "Front Yard"

Once thought to be merely an inert biological "glue" that held cells together, the material surrounding the cells, the extracellular matrix, is now understood to influence cellular development, movement, reproduction, and shape as well as biochemical function. Dr. Alfred Pischinger, professor of histology (the study of cell type and healthy cellular environment) and embryology at the University of Vienna, saw the importance of the extracellular matrix. In 1991 he wrote that the extracellular matrix is the support system for the cell and the foundation substance in which all cells are embedded.

The extracellular matrix is made up of collagens and polysaccharides that form proteoglycans. These two molecules form a water-filled, gel-like "ground substance" in which the connective tissue fibers are embedded. The condition of the space around a cell (its "front yard") and what happens there are as important to health as what occurs within the cell and in the membrane that encloses it.

How Toxins Deform the Extracellular Matrix   The extra-cellular matrix is prone to damage from both toxins and disease. The structure of this matrix gel controls blood circulation to the cells. As a tissue becomes diseased, the matrix thickens and loses fluidity, impeding the flow of nu-trients to the cells and the transport of cell waste products away from it. Toxins that have accumulated as a result of poor circulation are first deposited in this extracellular space. Diseases that change the gel matrix disturb circula-tion, providing a breeding ground for bacteria and other microbes. Diseases caused by toxicity commonly manifest in the spaces around cells rather than inside the cells. If condi-tions in this front-yard environment become too unfavor-able, seriously impeding normal oxygen and nutrient exchange and waste removal, cell function breaks down, and eventually cells die.

During detoxification therapy, it's important to increase the circulation through the lymph nodes.

When disease occurs, it is essential to reverse the ten-dency of the extracellular matrix to thicken and solidify. Un-fortunately, no conventional medical approaches or drug protocols are available that can reestablish a healthy extra-cellular matrix. However, it is very responsive to a variety of holistic therapies, such as acupuncture and massage. Be-cause the extracellular matrix is so susceptible to any type of change, even the delicate pinprick of an acupuncture needle can have a profound effect. These therapies can return the matrix to its normal, semiliquid state, increasing circulation to the cell so that toxic material can be carried away to the liver and kidneys for breakdown and removal. Many practitioners of alternative medicine realize that the basis of their efforts is to create a healthy extracellular matrix. In chapter 8 we'll go over several techniques, such as hydrotherapy and exercise, to stimulate circulation and normalize the extracellular space.

Vitamin C is critical in the assembly of connective tissue that surrounds cells. Vitamin C deficiency causes the extracellular matrix to become weak and fragile. That's one of the reasons vitamin C supplementation is an important part of our program. Health care management underestimates vitamin C's influence on our health as a stabilizer of collagen. Dr. Linus Pauling suggested that by improving the extracellular matrix, vitamin C prevents metastasis (the spread of cancer); it is this action that makes it an effective part of cancer therapy.

Blood: Aqua Vita, or the Water of Life

The blood links every organ in the body. It is made up of water, minerals, proteins, and a multitude of white and red blood cells. With each heartbeat, this water of life flows through all the tissues, delivering oxygen and critical nutrients to every cell and carting away metabolic debris. It also moves communication molecules from one part of the body to another, cleanses detoxification sites such as the liver, and provides a freeway along which designated antitoxin cells, such as those of the immune system, can travel. Your good health depends on the ability of the blood to perform these critical functions.

The blood is very sensitive to toxins, and it's the first of the body's fundamental building blocks to be affected by them. Once poisoned, the blood transports toxins to cells throughout the body. Blood can carry either the materials essential for health and healing or the elements that lead to disease and decay.

The primary aim of detoxification therapy is to clean the blood. The EcoTox program is built on this simple idea. We've found that changing and optimizing the diet and stimulating circulation encourage the organs of the immune system to filter the blood. As Dr. Harold Dick, N.D., said, "Our main job is to make over the blood. Until we do, we're just spinning our wheels." We believe that this unique concept, not commonly espoused in conventional medicine, will one day be recognized as the basis for healing by health care practitioners in a wide variety of disciplines.

Lymph: The Other Vital Fluid

After delivering nutrients and picking up cell waste, the blood travels by way of two routes. One route is through the arterial circulatory system. The other route is along the tiny tubules of the lymphatic system, a network of hair-thin capillaries that are present in virtually all tissues. Before entering this network, the blood is separated from red blood cells and small proteins, forming a clear fluid called lymph. The tiny tubules of the lymphatic system contain about 15 liters of lymph fluid, three times the amount of blood in the body.

The tubules empty into small filter areas called lymph nodes, found in the groin, armpits, neck, and throughout the abdomen surrounding the intestines. Lymph nodes, of which there are more than 600, act as filters. Inside each node, white blood cells stand guard, checking the lymphatic fluid for harmful bacterial, viral, and microbial material, much as airport x-ray machines scan the bags that pass through them for weapons. Once identified in the node, these "invaders" are labeled and ultimately destroyed. Lymphatic fluid reenters the bloodstream at the thoracic duct in the chest. Although blood undergoes a filtration process in the liver, the lymph nodes serve as a prefilter, screening out bacteria, viruses, and organic debris to prevent clogging and overloading in the liver.

Detoxification therapy is the ultimate form of natural protection. It's a method for rejuvenating the cellular soil.

A large portion of the lymphatic system resides inside the intestines, where many small nodes (Peyer's patches) are embedded in the tissue of the intestinal walls. At least 60 percent of the immune system is hidden in these nodes, which constitute what is known as gut-associated lymphoid tissue (GALT). It appears that most of the body's immune screening system is located here to facilitate the screening of all food and the potentially harmful "hitchhikers" that can accompany that food before it enters the bloodstream. Most of our daily immune function is made up of the complex interaction between diet, intestinal bacteria, and GALT. If there is inflammation in the intestines, this affects GALT.

GALT is also part of a communications network that links the intestines with the rest of the body, especially the brain. Highly active messenger molecules from the GALT send out "reports" about what we've eaten and how we are responding to it. This connection between the intestines and the brain demonstrates the importance of detoxification therapy in neurological, mental, and emotional health problems. It also supports the observation, long held by many parents of fussy, hungry children, that there's a direct cause-and-effect relationship between food and mood.

During detoxification therapy, it's important to increase the circulation through the lymph nodes. All of the exercises in the detoxification program aim to improve lymph circulation. Because lymphatic fluid flows upward, against gravity (the only exception being the fluid from the head and neck), its movement is accomplished through wavelike muscular contractions produced by vigorous, aerobic physical activity that pushes the fluid through the lymphatic channels.

Jumping on a minitrampoline for five to fifteen minutes daily or jumping rope are good activities for stimulating lymphatic circulation. Dry skin brushing—a simple do-it-yourself technique described in chapter 8 for stimulating the flow of lymphatic fluid—and inversion of the body also assist lymph drainage. The body can be therapeutically inverted by lying on gravity guidance boards or by doing the type of inversion poses included in yoga training exercises. Simply sitting so that the legs are higher than the pelvis encourages drainage from the legs into the nodes in the groin. Taking a few minutes a day to stretch the arms over the head helps move fluid through the nodes in the armpits. Hydrotherapy and massage can also increase lymphatic circulation.

Cells, blood, and lymph together comprise the "soil" of our inner microenvironment. The condition of this soil determines the status of our health. When the "soil" is nutrient rich and poison free, organs flourish and organ systems are strong. Chronic disease takes root when there is an imbalance in the cellular soil. Toxins are primarily responsible for polluting our cellular soil and undermining the ecological balance of our bodies. The prevalence of toxins in our day-to-day life means that none of us can completely escape from their effects. But many of the "insults" that create toxicity syndromes, which damage the cells, blood, and lymph (and impede their activities), are related to our lifestyle choices and dietary habits; these are factors you can control.

Now you know more about what "insults" your system, and you can make choices that help protect it. Detoxification therapy is the ultimate form of natural protection. It's a method for rejuvenating the cellular soil. And it's something you can choose to do for yourself and your health.

CHAPTER 4

The Six Steps of Detoxification

- **The Six Steps of Detoxification**
- **Step One: Remove the Obstacles to Health**
- **Step Two: Improve Circulation**

- **Step Three: Enhance Elimination**
- **Step Four: Repair the Gastrointestinal System**
- **Step Five: Stimulate the Liver**
- **Step Six: Transform Stress**

In the last chapter, you were introduced to the cellular environment of your body. In this chapter, you'll gain an understanding of the steps that constitute detoxification therapy, the principles on which those steps are based, and the ways in which those principles affect the cellular environment. Detoxification medicine is a multisystem approach that promotes health by stimulating optimum function in all the body's cells. It is a deceptively simple concept that makes a profound, positive, whole-body impact, an impact that cannot be duplicated by treatments that focus on only one part of the body or single health issues.

As a comprehensive health care strategy, a detoxification program like the one outlined in chapter 8 employs a variety of techniques to pull toxins out of the body, filter the blood, rehabilitate the intestinal tract, and improve digestion. This form of medicine is an expression of the principle "first do no harm," a tenet of the Hippocratic oath. It is noninvasive, safe, and remarkably effective for a variety of health problems and for most people. It is based on an understanding of the body's intrinsic capacity to rehabilitate and heal itself.

The Six Steps of Detoxification

The process of detoxification involves six steps that represent timeless and time-tested methods of self-healing—methods that work together to strengthen every tissue in the body and enhance the function of each of its systems. Our program fuses these steps together into a single, simple plan using diet and nutritional supplements, hydrotherapy (the use of hot and cold water to stimulate circulation), and exercise (see chapter 8). These steps are as follows:

1. Remove the obstacles to health

2. Improve circulation

3. Enhance elimination

4. Repair the gastrointestinal system

5. Stimulate the liver

6. Transform stress

The numbered steps listed previously are organized according to their importance in the process of detoxification. This means step 1, remove the obstacles to health, is the first priority of the program. Let's look at each of the six steps in detail.

Step One: Remove the Obstacles to Health

To remove obstacles to health and healing, you must first identify them. Our premise is that the main obstacle for most people today is the toxic strain that their bodies are under. An overload of unprocessed toxins impedes and causes disorder in normal metabolic function and undermines the natural mechanisms of protection and repair, creating barriers to wellness. Toxic exposure is the first obstacle that you must address, and the dietary component of the EcoTox program has been designed for this purpose.

Two days of liquids-only fasting and then a carefully planned five-day diet allow the digestive system to rest. Special supplements provide all the necessary nutrients to stimulate and support detoxification. Under these conditions, the body can dismantle the backlog of poisons in the tissues and concentrate its energy on healing.

Research has shown that a full-blown fast, consisting only of water or clear liquids and lasting more than a few days, actually hinders the process of detoxification, making it potentially harmful. Long fasts deplete concentrations of glutathione, an enzyme critical for protection against toxins. In addition, over time, all liquid fasts lower body stores of antioxidants, placing a person at risk for oxidative damage to critical organs that increases the rate of biological aging. Such fasts also supply little or no protein, and many of the liver's detoxifying processes depend on protein. High-protein

Case Histories

Roberta was a motivated business professional who decided to go through a detoxification program with a friend. She was forty-five, well muscled, and about 15 pounds overweight from too much food and not enough exercise. She was put on a rigorous seven-day program that included a period of fasting followed by a special diet, personal yoga training, acupuncture, massage, and lifestyle counseling. She discovered that detoxifying can be hard work. The rigor of waking up early in the morning, hard aerobic yoga training, controlled meals, and hardy living conditions at our retreat facility was a challenge for her, but she was determined to complete the program. After the week was over, she had lost weight, had more energy than when she started, and had acquired new and improved physical abilities. Although she hadn't been sick, the stimulation of her detoxification pathways made her feel remarkably better.

Julia was another person who benefited from detoxification. At age seventy-two, she suffered terrible pain from her arthritis, and her doctor had prescribed a number of powerful drugs. Because of her age and the barrage of drugs she was taking, some of which suppressed the immune system, the staff at our clinic was very concerned about her. We placed her on our diet and supplement program (in her condition, the exercises were too difficult for her). She followed this approach for one month and experienced remarkable results. Her color improved and she had a happier outlook on life. Most importantly, she was able to stop using her prescription painkillers because, after her detoxification, her arthritis symptoms had almost completely disappeared. Although you may not require detoxification for an entire month, after one week's worth you will feel much better.

diets increase the breakdown of xenobiotics (chemicals), which is why the EcoTox diet includes rice protein concentrates as part of its plan.

Removing the obstacles involves more than a few days of fasting. It also includes identifying those things in your life that could be contributing to your body's toxic burden. Perhaps the work you do exposes you to heavy metals or pesticides. You might have an allergic sensitivity to the foods you eat most often. Maybe something in your family situation is making you tense and anxious. Detoxification begins with a very thorough evaluation of all aspects of your life. You may find it helpful to consult a qualified health professional, who is a practitioner of detoxification medicine and skilled in guiding people through this analysis.

Step Two: Improve Circulation

Infection, inflammation, trauma, and disease processes respond positively to the enhanced circulation of blood and lymphatic fluid. The movement of these fluids brings nutrients, oxygen, and disease-fighting cells to damaged and distressed tissues and carries away metabolic waste, inflammatory by-products, and other toxins. As these fluids circulate, they are filtered in a continuous clean-and-flush operation. Defective circulation and stasis of the blood (stagnation from lack of movement) are the hallmarks of chronic and acute disease.

Chronic disorders of the sympathetic nervous system tend to be some of the major causes of poor circulation. The sympathetic nervous system is involved in regulating heart rate, breathing, and digestion. When the sympathetic nervous system is healthy, we experience an alert state of physical and mental well-being. This part of our nervous system is also responsible for our ability to react to sudden stresses, commonly known as our "fight or flight" response.

Overstimulation of the sympathetic nervous system from stress, injury, or shock is a common cause of poor circulation and poor health. Hyperactivity of the sympathetic nerves increases heart rate, slows digestion, increases respiration and metabolism, and can produce chronic, nagging sensations of fear and anxiety. Disorders of the sympathetic nervous system are not recognized in conventional medicine except in the form of severe diseases such as reflex sympathetic dystrophy. This syndrome often appears after a serious injury and has a wide variety of symptoms, including tenderness in the ends of the damaged extremity, burning pains, swelling, skin changes (such that the skin becomes thin, shiny, and cool), demineralization of the bone, increased sweating, and irreversible contraction of tendons and soft tissue structures. Another common outcome of too much sympathetic activity is Raynaud's disease, a syndrome characterized by inadequate blood circulation to the extremities.

Because hyperactivity in the sympathetic nervous system is not typically a recognized syndrome in conventional medicine, except in cases of shock and acute stress, few therapeutic remedies are available. Many patients who have this problem are mistakenly diagnosed with heart palpitations, anxiety disorders, or irritable bowel syndrome. However, hydrotherapy, acupuncture, manipulative therapies, and neural therapy have a significant and beneficial effect on the sympathetic nervous system, helping restore activity to normal. Because hydrotherapy is so effective in stimulating circulation, let's look at it in some detail.

Hydrotherapy

Encouraging the flow and filtering of blood and lymphatic fluid is the key to counteracting stasis (the stagnation of bodily fluids due to lack of movement), promoting detoxification, and jump-starting the immune system. Hydrotherapy, one of the oldest methods of encouraging proper circulation, entails the alternating use of brief applications of hot and cold water to drive blood to and from the skin's surface and encourage its flow through organ tissues. These applications can be either whole-body treatments or wet packs applied to specific areas. The method is simple, easy to do at home, and very effective at moving blood into areas of infection, congestion, swelling, inflammation, and irritation. As blood travels into and out of these areas, it delivers nutrients and carries away cellular waste products and other toxic substances.

Detoxification is noninvasive, safe, and remarkably effective for a variety of health problems and for most people. It is based on an understanding of the body's intrinsic capacity to rehabilitate and heal itself.

Naturopathic physicians, who first began to practice in the United States at the turn of the twentieth century, were typically trained in Europe at the great health spas. There they learned to use special diets and the application of hot and cold water packs in specific sequences to certain body parts to treat cancer, tuberculosis, chronic infections, and many other serious diseases. The stimulation of blood circulation with hydrotherapy enhances the activity of the immune system by increasing the number of white blood cells, the rate of white blood cell movement, and the activity and success rate of white blood cells in killing germs. Such simple remedies, however, are no longer in fashion, despite the fact that they have far fewer side effects than many drug therapies currently in use and can be equally effective. Although the effectiveness of such treatment is often ignored by conventional medicine, its power should not be underestimated. In our clinic, we have seen hydrotherapy turn around many very sick patients.

In chapter 8, we'll discuss how to use three forms of hot and cold water therapy to improve circulation: the shower method, bath and wet sheet method, and alternating applications of hot and cold packs. Sauna sessions, which promote sweating, followed by cold water washing constitute a fourth but slightly different form of hydrotherapy.

Hydrotherapy stimulates reflex points on the skin's surface. A reflex point is a specific location on the outside of the body that is related to a specific organ inside the body (see figure 4.1). Stimulating the reflex point improves the flow of blood to and from the corresponding organ. There are, for example, reflex points in the feet for the uterus. For thousands of years, Chinese acupuncture has taught the relationship of points on the feet to the prostate, bladder, uterus, and ovaries. An old "trick" to stop uterine hemorrhaging was to put the feet of the bleeding woman into ice-cold water.

When the reflex points corresponding to organs of detoxification, such as the liver and intestines, are stimulated, the increased circulation through these areas enhances the filtering and cleaning of the blood.

Step Three: Enhance Elimination

Once the circulatory system has begun moving poisons from toxic tissues, the body must eliminate them via sweat, urine, and feces. Elimination is enhanced by strengthening and

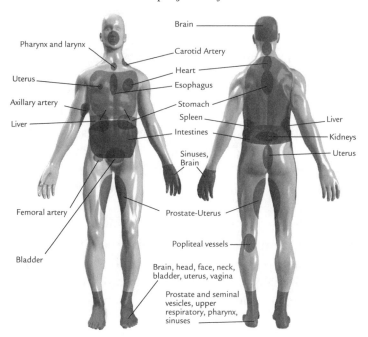

Figure 4.1.

Reflex points of the skin.

opening the avenues of excretion: the sweat glands in the skin, the kidneys, and the intestines. There are various ways we can increase the removal of toxins through these exits: purgation through colonic irrigation, herbal laxatives, and vitamin C colon flushes for the intestines; diuresis (increased therapeutic urination) for the kidneys; and diaphoresis (sweating therapy) for the skin. All of these techniques increase the filtering and elimination of toxic body fluids.

In your seven-day program, a brief fast plus a high intake of fiber, charcoal, and vitamin C helps to clear the colon; a high intake of purified fluids flushes the kidneys; and hydrotherapy, exercise, and saunas promote sweating. Cathartics are also recommended for those who are constipated. The following sections explain the therapies for the intestines, kidneys, and skin.

The Intestines

Because of the interrelationship between immune function and the intestines, it makes sense that cleansing them has a powerful disease-modifying effect. In addition, the liver cleanses the blood of most poisons, which are then excreted into the bile (a fat-dissolving digestive enzyme), which squirts into the intestines during digestion. Bile, and the toxins that it contains, is incorporated into the stool. When the stool doesn't move through the intestines easily and relatively quickly, waste products accumulate and clog the bowel, which irritates the delicate lining of the large intestine, allowing waste products and other toxins to be reabsorbed into the bloodstream. Waste remaining in contact with the intestinal wall for an abnormally long period of time can cause chronic inflammation and other serious complications.

The process of detoxification involves timeless and time-tested methods of self-healing—methods that work together to strengthen every tissue in the body and enhance the function of each of its systems.

Normal bowel transit time (the number of hours between eating food and excreting the waste products) ranges from twenty to forty-eight hours. However, for many people in Western society, transit time is two, three, or even five times longer. Bowel movements among those eating a typical American diet are significantly lighter and smaller in volume than those of people in many third-world nations who consume diets higher in fiber. It is also interesting to note that cancer is almost nonexistent among people in these cultures.

The urge to have a bowel movement should occur about twenty minutes after eating, a sort of an out-with-the-old, in-with-the-new reflex. Ideally, this should happen after every meal, as it does in infants, and anything less frequent than once a day constitutes constipation. Cow's milk and the products made from it are a major cause of chronic constipation because they can cause an allergic reaction and lectin agglutination (an excess of mucus, which has a tendency to bind the stool). (For a complete discussion of the effects of eating the wrong type of dietary lectins, see *Eat Right for Your Type* by Peter D'Adamo.)

Some clinics and practitioners that specialize in detoxification therapy emphasize the need for colon washing, also called colonic irrigation, colon hydrotherapy, or enemas. Colonic irrigation is not included in the EcoTox program because we find it to be unnecessary if the program is followed in its entirety. However, this doesn't mean that colonics aren't helpful. They are documented to be effective, and some of our patients are avid fans of this treatment.

For those who are constipated (and for fever, infections, and inflammation), we recommend purgation therapy using an herbal cathartic. The formula detailed in chapter 8 is one advocated by Dr. O. G. Carroll, a renowned naturopathic physician. The combination of *Artemisia absinthum* and cape aloe is taken as a capsule, once a day, to flush the intestines. Dr. Carroll prescribes this cathartic at the beginning of a cold, during a healing crisis, or at any time when the bowels do not empty smoothly. This is a strong purgative, so it shouldn't be used on a daily basis.

High doses of vitamin C flush provide another good way to improve bowel transit time while simultaneously providing antioxidant protection for the immune system. This is especially important when dangerous toxins are being excreted in the bile. This method is helpful, for example, for people who are having their mercury amalgam dental fillings removed. In high doses, vitamin C inactivates any toxins in the intestines as they pass out through the stool, and we have found that there is a lower incidence of healing crises in people taking high doses during detoxification (for more on the benefits of vitamin C, see chapter 8). For people suffering from constipation, incorporating a dose of vitamin C daily may bring wonderful results.

The Kidneys

Promoting the flow of toxins through the kidneys requires adequate fluid intake. Dehydration, or a lack of adequate water intake, is a common symptom in many of our patients. The body loses an amazing 1 pint of fluid per hour through sweating (which isn't always obvious), and it's easy to forget to replace this fluid. Dehydration results in an accumulation of harmful substances in the blood that act on cell membranes and have an adverse effect on the kidneys, nervous system, and immune system.

Diuresis is a way to increase the flow of fluid through the kidneys. During detoxification, simply drinking 2 liters of pure, filtered water daily is sufficient for diuresis and the removal of toxins. You need to drink extra water when undergoing any sweating therapy (for example, saunas), when temperatures are excessively high, and before and after exercise.

The Skin

The skin acts like a second kidney. Sweat glands permeate the skin's 11,000 square feet of surface area (which includes skin surface, sweat glands, and ducts). These glands are a major thoroughfare for the elimination of toxins. Fluids in

The Benefits of Sweating Therapy

Two studies found that sweating reversed brain dysfunction in firefighters poisoned by industrial toxins. Treatment programs involved physical exercise for twenty to thirty minutes, a 140- to 180-degree sauna for two and a half hours, and a vitamin program consisting of vitamins C, A, D, E, and B-complex; the minerals calcium, magnesium, iron, zinc, manganese, copper, potassium, and iodine; and a supplement of essential fatty acids. After three weeks on this program, participants showed improvement on intelligence tests, indicating that the toxins were eliminated and thus no longer causing brain dysfunction.

the blood and lymph are "sacrificed" to manufacture sweat. When we sweat, some of the poisons these fluids contain are excreted through the skin. As much as 30 percent of the body's blood supply is held in the skin's peripheral blood vessels (that is, those near the surface of the skin), and up to 60 percent of the blood supply can enter when the skin is heated. Sweating intensively, a person can lose as much as 3 liters (or about 8 pounds) of fluid per hour, making diaphoresis, or sweating therapy, very effective for removing toxins from the body.

The body stores many toxins in fatty tissue. Sweating therapy reduces fat stores quickly, releasing these poisons for excretion through the stimulation of receptors in the fat. Tissue biochemistry and nervous system functioning undergo changes in sauna therapy, activating fat stores and facilitating fat loss. In fact, detoxification is probably one of the healthiest ways to reduce fat and lose weight. The use of a special diet, supplements, and sweating therapy provides a fast exit for excess bulk and fat-soluble toxins that are stored in the body. Although not meant as a weight-loss system, you'll discover that most of the clinical secrets for helping shed difficult pounds are found in our program. Almost all our patients lose 7 to 14 pounds in one to two weeks, and, because they stay on a maintenance program, the weight does not come back.

Increasing your body temperature (not exceeding 104 degrees Fahrenheit, which could be dangerous) also creates a more favorable climate for immune system activity. During sweating therapy, immune reactions increase because white blood cells move more easily into the skin.

Step Four: Repair the Gastrointestinal System

Home to a fantastic array of microbial species whose numbers exceed the total number of cells in the body, the gastrointestinal (GI) system is an incredibly complex system. At least four hundred species of microorganisms exist in the human GI tract, amounting to about 3 pounds of bacteria. Some of these are beneficial, some are dangerous, and both compete for dominance. In a healthy system, the good bacteria outnumber the bad and keep the size of the unwholesome population in check.

When allowed to outnumber good bacteria, bad bacteria produce dangerous toxins that are absorbed into the bloodstream and are associated with a host of acute and chronic diseases, including rheumatoid arthritis, colitis, diabetes, meningitis, myasthenia gravis, Grave's disease, Hashimoto's thyroiditis, and bowel cancer. Imbalances between the good and bad bacteria in the intestines have also been linked to food allergies; skin conditions such as eczema, psoriasis, acne, and urticaria (hives); migraine headaches; ankylosing spondylitis (rheumatoid arthritis of the spine);

systemic lupus erythematosis; ulcerative colitis; Crohn's disease; otitis media (ear inflammation); sinusitis; asthma; premature labor and delivery; peptic ulcers; premenstrual syndrome; and cystitis.

Many activities take place simultaneously in the 22 feet of tubing that make up the digestive and intestinal tract: the breakdown of food, scanning of the food by the immune system, detoxification of poorly digested fermented toxins, filtering of food and intestinal bacteria, and elimination. The normal cycling of substances in and out of your system depends on the integrity of the membrane that keeps the intestinal tract's contents separate from the rest of the body and on the maintenance of a precise bacterial and chemical environment. The root cause of many health problems can be traced back to poor GI system functioning, and what happens here can affect the entire body. For example, an imbalance in the intestinal ecosystem can allow harmful bacteria and yeast to multiply uncontrollably; injure the membranes that line the intestines, allowing undigested food products and other contaminants to leak into the bloodstream; alter detoxification ability; and lead to the production of dangerous chemicals.

Sources of Intestinal Toxins

An overabundance of dangerous microbial intestinal bacteria can result from the repeated use of antibiotics. Antibiotic therapy upsets the natural balance of bacteria in the intestines by indiscriminately killing off both beneficial and pathogenic microbes. Supplementing with *Lactobacillus acidophilus* and *L. bifidus* is an effective way to prevent the side effects of antibiotic therapy (for more information about reseeding the intestines with *Lactobacillus acidophilus* and *L. bifidus,* see chapter 8). Other factors that disturb the normal balance of bacteria in the GI system include steroid drugs, pregnancy, birth control pills or estrogen replacement therapy (ERT), insufficient hydrochloric acid in the stomach, slow bowel transit time, inadequate intake of dietary fiber, poor immune function, and diabetes.

Some bacteria in the GI system produce endotoxins, which are substances that have the capacity to cause cell membrane destruction in a process called peroxidation. This process is equivalent to a molecular forest fire, and only antioxidants can put it out. Unchecked, lipid peroxidation can start a chain reaction that results in massive cellular damage. High levels of endotoxins create a free-radical toxicity syndrome and cause premature aging, alterations to DNA, carcinogenesis, changes in cell membranes, cell death, and oxidative destruction of red blood cells. People who have food and environmental sensitivities might be suffering from endotoxemia.

Bacterial fermentation creates another group of toxins (amines, indoles, and skatols from putrefying intestinal contents) that can be measured in elevated quantities in the urine of individuals who have poor digestion and poor bowel function. When there is excessive sugar in the diet, yeasts in the GI system cause it to ferment, producing toxic chemicals called aldehydes.

The foods that we eat also generate intestinal toxins. All charbroiled meats have heterocyclic compounds that are converted into carcinogens by GI system bacteria. Molds breed on certain nuts and grains that produce carcinogens such as aflatoxin, one of the most dangerous cancer-causing substances known to man. When people with sensitivities to wheat, corn, and dairy products eat foods containing these ingredients, their immune systems react by releasing chemicals in the bloodstream, which upset their health. Chronic headaches, sore throats, and respiratory infections are extremely common examples of symptoms caused by intestinal food allergies.

Parasites that set up house in the GI system constitute another source of toxicity. The life cycle activity of these invading organisms irritates the intestinal lining, causing chronic inflammation and intestinal permeability.

Intestinal Permeability (Leaky Gut Syndrome)

If the contents of the bowel are not eliminated and instead remain in the intestines, or if food allergies cause immune reactions, the intestinal membranes become irritated and inflamed. This can lead to damage of the delicate intestinal lining, creating tiny cracks and microscopic holes that allow toxins to pass through into the circulating blood. Figure 4.2 illustrates how toxins can seep into these holes. The leakage of bacterial toxins, undigested food molecules, and other toxins from the bowel into the bloodstream— called intestinal permeability, or leaky gut syndrome— contributes significantly to detoxification problems in the liver. These detoxification problems accelerate aging and can cause a predisposition to other diseases. Intestinal permeability is commonly seen in patients who have Crohn's disease, food allergies, celiac disease, rheumatoid arthritis, and schizophrenia.

Normally, the food we eat is digested, detoxified, screened by our immune system, and eventually absorbed through the intestinal lining. However, only nutrient-sized molecules are supposed to pass through this lining and into the bloodstream. This is called selective permeability. When the selective permeability of the intestinal membrane is lost because localized inflammation has undermined the integrity of the membrane's surface, the barrier between the bowels and the rest of the body is compromised; material meant to be eliminated can pollute the sterile environment of the bloodstream, wreaking havoc on immune function and all organs of the body. Toxins entering the bloodstream from the intestines clog up the detoxifying mechanisms in the liver, making us more vulnerable to further harm from other toxins in the environment.

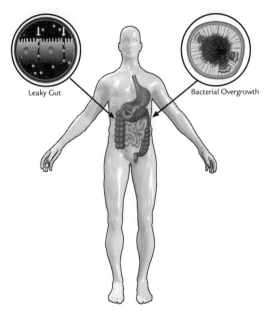

Figure 4.2

Small holes in the intestinal lining due to chronic irritation allow
toxins to slip into the bloodstream. Overgrowth of harmful bacteria in the gastrointestinal tract can produce toxins. Such conditions create more detoxification work for the liver.

Many factors can cause the intestinal lining to break
down. Excessive inflammation in the bowel sets off the process
by destroying the membrane filter. If the condition persists, it
can cause as much as a sixfold increase in intestinal permeability. Some common causes of inflammation are poorly digested
foods, excessive alcohol intake, and food allergens.

Many people who can't properly digest wheat react to
it as an allergen. In those who have a wheat or gluten allergy,
the intestinal lining breaks down as a result of chronic inflammation due to the allergic reaction to wheat. Important
transport sites involved in the absorption of protein and
mineral molecules from the gut are also destroyed, leading
to deficiencies of these essential nutrients. Wheat- or gluten-

Healing Strategies

Research performed by Jeff Bland, Ph.D., a nutritional biochemist and president of Healthcomm Inc. (www.healthcomm.com) in Gig Harbor, Washington, shows that to repair the GI system and enhance its detoxification mechanism a complete program must include all of the following strategies:

1. Reseed the intestines with friendly bacteria.

2. Improve digestion so food is properly processed and does not putrefy.

3. Increase bowel transit time.

4. Implement practices that, over time, act to minimize intestinal permeability.

The EcoTox program utilizes a carefully planned diet that eliminates irritants, gives the GI system a rest, and uses nutrient support and hydrotherapy to achieve all these goals.

sensitive individuals who have followed our diet, which eliminates this inflammatory food and all products made with it, have had their intestines begin to heal within a week.

In addition, intestinal infections cause and increase permeability. We have seen patients in our clinic, for example, who suddenly developed food allergies after salmonella infections. This is probably why chronic health symptoms can develop for some patients after a serious intestinal infection. Drugs can increase intestinal permeability as well. Aspirin and nonsteroidal anti-inflammatory drugs (NSAIDs) are the worst offenders. The regular use of anti-inflammatory drugs is a major source of irritation to the bowel lining and can lead to the destruction of the intestinal barrier. Unfortunately, those who have osteoarthritis—who are most likely to use NSAIDs—are the least likely to be able to tolerate increased intestinal permeability. These people also usually have food allergies. The NSAIDs they take to cope with the pain of osteoarthritis increase the leakage of food antigens (chemicals released due to the allergic reaction) into their bloodstream, which aggravates their disease condition.

As we age, intestinal permeability tends to increase. Fortunately, increasing our intake of dietary fiber as we age can offset damage to the intestines.

Step Five: Stimulate the Liver

The liver is the body's master modification site. It is responsible for a process called biotransformation. As blood passes through the liver with a load of raw materials, toxins are scavenged, neutralized, and reassembled for elimination; food nutrients are chemically prepared for conversion to energy; vitamins A, D, and B_{12} and the mineral iron are "tagged" for storage or distribution; and compounds necessary for cell formation and repair, digestion, and the manufacture of hormones are produced. The liver creates bile and cholesterol, which are essential for the proper utilization and disposal of dietary fats. In fact, almost all metabolic activity and systemic function can be linked in some way to the liver. Therefore, if this organ is not operating at full capacity, the effects will resonate throughout the body.

Because of the way in which most of us eat and live, the liver can be overburdened, sluggish, and congested. Constant exposure to a wide variety of toxins and contaminants; unhealthy, nutrient-poor diets high in saturated and hydrogenated fats; and a leaky gut are among the primary causes of liver burnout. Resuscitating the liver is a vital step in the process of detoxification. Diet, herbs, nutrients, exercise, and hydrotherapy help to stimulate the liver's activity and move accumulated toxins out with the bile.

Detoxification begins with a very thorough evaluation of all aspects of your life.

Because detoxification is such a nutrient-demanding process, fasting and diet must be structured properly. We promote the use of amino acids to drive detoxification; antioxidants, other vitamins, and herbs to assist the process, prevent free-radical damage, and protect the liver and other organs from the biochemical fireworks that go off during detoxification reactions; and herbs to stimulate the production of bile so that the toxins can be carried away from the liver. We've used this approach in our clinic for more than ten years. For long-term health maintenance, we suggest continuing a similar program of supplementation after your detoxification week to keep your liver working at top performance every day.

In addition, special circulation-enhancing practices, such as hydrotherapy and saunas, jumping rope, and yoga, are used to force the movement of blood through the intestines and liver, causing an increase in immune and detoxification function. Without the enhanced circulation, the liver will not clean the blood as effectively. Although no medical research validates the use of enhanced circulation for detoxification, except for saunas, our clinical experience has shown excellent results with this essential part of the program.

Step Six: Transform Stress

For thousands of years, physicians have watched their patients respond to therapies with a wide range of results. Some recover fully, whereas others with identical diseases and treatment protocols fail to improve. As we discussed earlier in chapter 1, the mind is part of both the cause and the cure of many diseases. It's also a variable that's often overlooked in clinical care. A person can receive the best available medical evaluation and treatment, but the chances for a successful recovery decrease if the diagnosis and the therapeutic interaction don't alleviate stress, promote relaxation, and stimulate positive feelings of hope, faith, and trust.

Many examples can be found in medical literature, both old and new, that attest to the relationship between health, emotions (the mind), and therapeutic results. Ancient Chinese medical texts explain that stress in the form of worry upsets the digestive system, stress from fear disturbs kidney function, stress from anger and frustration injures the liver's ability to clean and circulate the blood, and stress from grief damages the lungs, causing susceptibility to respiratory infections.

The effects of negativity and stress on health and healing have been observed and reported by contemporary researchers as well. These researchers in psychosomatic medicine were on the forefront of mind-body medicine in the early part of the twentieth century. For example, Dr. Walter Cannon of Harvard Medical School wrote about what he called "voodoo death," the practice, common in many indigenous third-world cultures, of killing a member of the community by placing a curse on them: "The suggestion that I offer . . . is that 'voodoo death' may be real, and that it may be explained as due to shocking emotional stress—to obvious or repressed terror."

This statement reveals Dr. Cannon's understanding of the profound effect that the mind, through belief, can exert on the trillions of cells that make up the body. Other studies have shown that negative emotional states and stressful circumstances prompt a fight-or-flight response that triggers a broad array of electrochemical activity. The results are physical changes that have been linked to immune function.

Detoxification is probably one of the healthiest ways to reduce fat and lose weight.

The current model for explaining how emotions, mood, and psychological stress interact involves the cerebral-limbic-hypothalamic axis in the brain. According to psychiatrist Ernest Rossi, M.D., "The hypothalamus is thus the major output pathway of the limbic system. It integrates the sensory-perceptual, emotional, and cognitive function of the mind with the biology of the body." This axis translates stress and anxiety into a stress-hormone response. These hormones suppress the function of the immune system.

Over time these stress hormones can upset every organ system in the body. For example, one study showed that stress hormones blocked the liver's ability to detoxify an anti-inflammatory drug, leaving it to circulate as unprocessed poison. Stress chemicals produced in the body can be extremely destructive. The oxidation of the stress hormone adrenaline forms a substance called adrenochrome, which affects both the cardiovascular and nervous systems. High serum concentrations of oxidized adrenaline (in the form of adrenochrome) can damage the heart, resulting in coronary spasm, heart arrhythmia, ultrastructural heart damage, and ventricular dysfunction.

Stress upsets the body's detoxification systems and weakens the body's natural filtering mechanisms, increasing intestinal permeability. By altering intestinal permeability, stress not only increases the liver's workload but also threatens the delicate environment of the central nervous system. Just as the intestines are supposed to maintain a protective separation between their contents and the bloodstream, the blood-brain barrier is supposed to prevent certain substances in the blood from passing into the brain. Stress contributes to the permeability of the blood-brain barrier.

Negative thinking alters cardiovascular function, too. For example, it has been clearly established that even low levels of stress trigger the onset of myocardial ischemia (decreased blood flow to the heart, which signals the beginning of a heart attack). Hypertension and coronary artery disease have been linked to stress as well.

By striving to replace negative emotions and thoughts with positive ones, the mind is purified of subtle toxins that eventually create biochemical toxins in the bloodstream.

The newly emerging field of psychoneuroimmunology explores the precise relationship between mind and body. Researchers have been able to verify that mental and emotional states have the ability to affect the production of hormones and neurotransmitters (the so-called feel-good brain chemicals), affect the body's detoxification pathways, and influence treatment outcomes. It is believed that steroids, catecholamines (stress hormones), neuropeptides, and endorphins are the biochemical language produced in the body from stress.

These stress-related changes in biochemistry translate into depression, negative emotions, and diseases of the immune and central nervous systems. Medical research on detoxification has focused mainly on the effect of environmental toxins on the liver, the immune system, and the brain. However, stress can also be a toxin. Anger, jealousy, sadness, grief, and self-recrimination can also impact detoxification enzymes and contribute to measurable toxicity syndromes.

Your health care regimen must address the toxicity of the mind. We've found that generating positive emotions is the most important key to detoxifying the mind. Changing your thoughts to focus on the positive can be done effectively with self-hypnosis, prayer, affirmations, and altering the home or work environments so that the same habits of negative thought are unlikely to occur. Daily relaxation through hobbies, reading, playing music, exercise, and adequate rest are only a few of the important activities that protect us from mental agitation and physical stress.

In chapter 8 we'll review a set of recommended breath-training and relaxation exercises that are designed to regulate the nervous system and reduce the damaging effects of stress. By striving to replace negative emotions and thoughts with positive ones, the mind is purified of subtle toxins that eventually create biochemical toxins in the bloodstream.

Because the liver plays such a vital role in detoxification, the next chapter is devoted to a discussion of its various specialized functions. It's impossible to grasp the value of the EcoTox program without first understanding the liver's role in detoxification.

CHAPTER 5

The Liver

Your Detoxification Powerhouse

- **The Liver: Source of Transformation**
- **The Liver's Detoxification Function**
- **Problems in Phase 1 and Phase 2 Detoxification**
- **The Gallbladder, Bile, and Gallstones**
- **Detoxification and You**

M ost of the biochemical activity of detoxification takes place in the gastrointestinal system and the liver. And it is the liver, our largest single organ, that is primarily responsible for screening every molecule that circulates in the body and transforming those that are toxic into harmless "biodegradable" substances. It cleans and purifies the blood that nourishes the entire body. Any weakness or debility of the liver impacts every other organ system. One of the basic tenets of naturopathic medicine is that many diseases can be treated by enhancing liver function. Current scientific and medical research has begun to verify the reasoning behind the clinical approach of natural physicians. In this chapter, we'll show you how this detoxification powerhouse works to keep you healthy.

The Liver: Source of Transformation

The liver is a dense, football-sized filtering and processing plant that sits under your ribs on the right side of your abdomen. It is a collection of different types of cells with different jobs, ranging from the conversion of food into compounds the body can use to the breakdown of heavy metals, poisonous agricultural chemicals, and metabolic byproducts (see figure 5.1). The liver performs approximately five hundred distinct functions, more than any other organ in the body. It issues numerous biochemical orders to other organs and systems. Some of its main duties include:

Carbohydrate metabolism. Stores sugars, converts different types of sugars into glucose, and maintains blood sugar levels.

Fat metabolism. Produces bile, which makes dietary fats digestible; breaks down fats so they can be used to fuel metabolic activity; manufactures triglycerides, lipoproteins, and cholesterol; and converts carbohydrates and proteins into useable energy forms.

Protein metabolism. Breaks down protein and restructures it to be used in the production of other compounds the body needs.

Storage of nutrients. Stores vitamins D, A, and B_{12} and the mineral iron.

Immune defense center. Filters the blood, removing harmful bacteria, viruses, toxins, yeast, and other foreign substances.

Conversion of hormones, metabolic waste products, toxins, and other destructive substances. Dismantles and alters the molecular structure of unwanted and unhealthy materials so that they can be eliminated.

Is Your Liver Healthy?

Medical doctors use a group of blood tests to look for liver damage in cases of infectious liver disease and alcoholic liver disease, but these tests are not effective in showing the liver's functional capability. Functional capability refers to the liver's capacity for performance. Loss of functional capability might not show up in conventional liver–blood screening tests, but naturopathic physicians identify the condition, and the attendant slowdown in detoxification, as a "sluggish liver." Signs of a sluggish liver are sallow skin color and poor skin tone, dark circles under the eyes, a yellow-coated tongue, a bitter taste in the mouth, headaches, irritability, premenstrual tension, arthritis, and inability to digest fats (recognizable as indigestion after eating high-fat meals). There are also tests you can order from several labs that, along with a medical checkup, can assess your liver's functional capability (for more details, see chapter 7).

One of the basic tenets of naturopathic medicine is that many diseases can be treated by enhancing liver function.

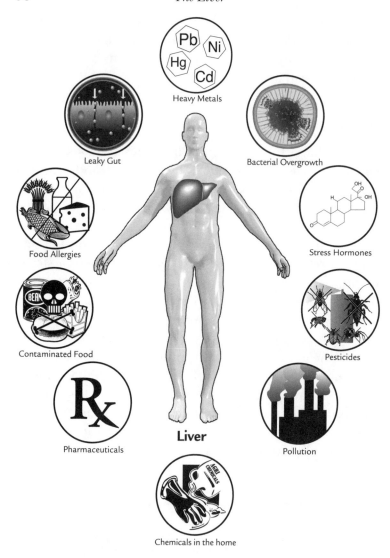

Figure 5.1: The Liver

The liver fights to cleanse your body of toxins, some of which are
environmental, and others that are produced within your own body.

Even when the liver is sluggish, it is able to do much of
its most important work. That's because there are six detoxification pathways in the liver, and they have the ability to

back up and cover for one another. This is called *functional reserve,* which allows the liver to continue to operate even after injury, inflammation, or illness has destroyed as much as 80 to 90 percent of its ability to function. Poor digestion, poor nutrition, poor excretion of bile, genetic weakness, and excessive exposure to toxins impair liver function and contribute to the depletion of its functional reserves. A human being cannot survive more than twenty-four hours without a functioning liver. To protect and care for this indispensable organ, you must first understand the liver's role in the process of molecular purification and transformation. Your health depends on it.

The Liver's Detoxification Function

Your body doesn't like to keep any molecules around for a long time. Even "good" molecules, such as hormones, are constantly being disassembled and reconstructed to prepare them to be recycled or eliminated. Thanks to detoxification enzymes, the liver is able to break up most molecules, even toxic and dangerous ones. Enzymes are molecules that act as catalysts in the transformation process. There are thousands of different enzymes, each with a unique role.

Think of this detoxification process as a two-phase wash cycle. Enzymes are like the soap that liberates grease into little droplets, removing impurities that the water can't remove on its own. In the first part of the wash cycle (Phase 1), enzymes break toxins down into intermediate forms. Figure 5.2 illustrates the complicated process of how some common toxins are broken down during Phase 1 detoxification. Some toxins are ready for elimination at this stage, but others require a second wash cycle. In Phase 2, these intermediate compounds are routed along one of six chemically driven detoxification pathways, where they are further broken down, and then bound to specific types of protein molecules

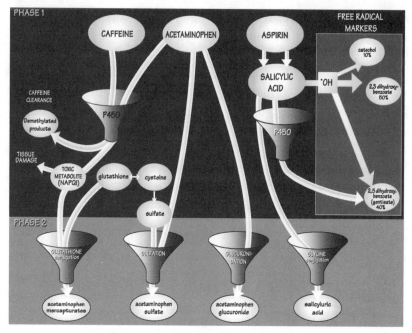

Figure 5.2 Phase 1 and Phase 2 Detoxification

Inside the liver a variety of enzymes break down toxins
through a number of chemical reactions. These new broken-down toxins
are then ready for Phase 2 detoxification.

that act as "escorts" to guide them out of the body, allowing
them to exit through the kidneys (in the form of urine) or
the bile (in the form of feces). This process is called conjugation and is illustrated in figure 5.3. Of the six pathways, three
warrant special mention.

One of the most important systems in Phase 2 is the
glutathione conjugation pathway, which utilizes glutathione
for the detoxification of deadly industrial toxins such as
PCBs and the breakdown of carcinogens. Its activity accounts
for up to 60 percent of the toxins excreted in the bile. Glutathione also circulates through the bloodstream combating
free radicals. No other conjugating substance is as versatile
as glutathione and the body's supply of it, most of which is

Detoxification—*Bio-Reactive Mechanisms*
Phase II Pathways

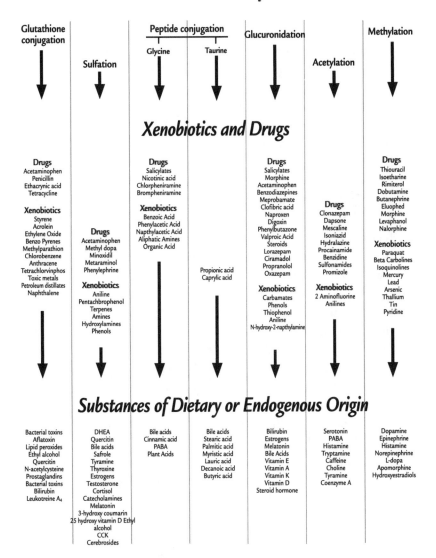

Xenobiotics and Drugs

Glutathione conjugation

Drugs
Acetaminophen
Penicillin
Ethacrynic acid
Tetracycline

Xenobiotics
Styrene
Acrolein
Ethylene Oxide
Benzo Pyrenes
Methylparathion
Chlorobenzene
Anthracene
Tetrachlorvinphos
Toxic metals
Petroleum distillates
Naphthalene

Sulfation

Drugs
Acetaminophen
Methyl dopa
Minoxidil
Metaraminol
Phenylephrine

Xenobiotics
Aniline
Pentachbrophenol
Terpenes
Amines
Hydroxylamines
Phenols

Peptide conjugation

Glycine

Drugs
Salicylates
Nicotinic acid
Chlorpheniramine
Brompheniramine

Xenobiotics
Benzoic Acid
Phenylacetic Acid
Napthylacetic Acid
Aliphatic Amines
Organic Acid

Taurine

Propionic acid
Caprylic acid

Glucuronidation

Drugs
Salicylates
Morphine
Acetaminophen
Benzodiazepines
Meprobamate
Clofibric acid
Naproxen
Digoxin
Phenylbutazone
Valproic Acid
Steroids
Lorazepam
Ciramadol
Propranolol
Oxazepam

Xenobiotics
Carbamates
Phenols
Thiophenol
Aniline
N-hydroxy-2-napthylamine

Acetylation

Drugs
Clonazepam
Dapsone
Mescaline
Isoniazid
Hydralazine
Procainamide
Benzidine
Sulfonamides
Promizole

Xenobiotics
2 Aminofluorine
Anilines

Methylation

Drugs
Thiouracil
Isotharine
Rimiterol
Dobutamine
Butanephrine
Eluophed
Morphine
Levaphanol
Nalorphine

Xenobiotics
Paraquat
Beta Carbolines
Isoquinolines
Mercury
Lead
Arsenic
Thallium
Tin
Pyridine

Substances of Dietary or Endogenous Origin

Bacterial toxins
Aflatoxin
Lipid peroxides
Ethyl alcohol
Quercitin
N-acetylcysteine
Prostaglandins
Bacterial toxins
Bilirubin
Leukotreine A₄

DHEA
Quercitin
Bile acids
Safrole
Tyramine
Thyroxine
Estrogens
Testosterone
Cortisol
Catecholamines
Melatonin
3-hydroxy coumarin
25 hydroxy vitamin D Ethyl
alcohol
CCK
Cerebrosides

Bile acids
Cinnamic acid
PABA
Plant Acids

Bile acids
Stearic acid
Palmitic acid
Myristic acid
Lauric acid
Decanoic acid
Butyric acid

Bilirubin
Estrogens
Melatonin
Bile Acids
Vitamin E
Vitamin A
Vitamin K
Vitamin D
Steroid hormone

Serotonin
PABA
Histamine
Tryptamine
Caffeine
Choline
Tyramine
Coenzyme A

Dopamine
Epinephrine
Histamine
Norepinephrine
L-dopa
Apomorphine
Hydroxyestradiols

Figure 5.3 Phase 2 Detoxification

This diagram illustrates which of the different pathways within Phase 2 detoxification break down both chemicals outside the body (xenobiotics and drugs) and those formed within the body (substances of dietary or endogenous origin).

produced by the liver, is easily depleted. Exposure to high levels of toxins exhausts reserves of glutathione, possibly increasing susceptibility to cancer. Chronic disease, HIV, and cirrhosis use up reserves of glutathione. Excessive exercise, which increases oxidative stress and free-radical production, and alcohol consumption, which blocks glutathione production, also deplete glutathione in the blood.

The weakest pathway in most people, from a dietary standpoint, is sulfation, the one responsible for the transformation of neurotransmitters, steroid hormones, drugs, industrial chemicals, phenolics (compounds derived from benzene, commonly used in plastics, disinfectants, and pharmaceuticals), and especially toxins from intestinal bacteria and the environment. Intake of too little dietary sulfur, a molecule that must come from our diets, is a cause of ineffective detoxification. If your exposure to substances that need to be detoxified via the sulfation pathway is high, but your sulfate reserves are low due to an inadequate diet, you will not be able to break down these toxins.

Studies have established a strong association between the function of the sulfation pathway and a variety of illnesses including Alzheimer's disease, Parkinson's disease, motor neuron disease, autism, primary biliary cirrhosis, rheumatoid arthritis, food sensitivity, and multiple chemical sensitivity. The detoxification profile test described in chapter 7 identifies alterations in this pathway.

The body manufactures five different types of amino acids that form a third detoxification pathway: glycine, taurine, glutamine, arginine, and ornithine. Of these, glycine is the most important for the neutralization of toxins. In some cases, the body cannot make enough glycine to keep up with its own detoxification needs. Though not considered an essential amino acid because the body can make it, glycine production depends on an adequate intake of dietary protein. Individuals who eat a protein-deficient diet have trouble detoxifying environmental pollutants.

Glycine supplies can be depleted by lifestyle stresses. Benzoates, for example, found in soft drinks, bind with glycine and rob the body's store of it. One study found that people who consumed a large number of soft drinks had problems breaking down toluene, a common industrial organic solvent. Aspirin also slows down this detoxification pathway because it competes for available glycine in the liver. When the diet is supplemented with glycine, as well as the other nonessential amino acids, there is a noticeable improvement in the detoxification capabilities of many people.

Problems in Phase 1 and Phase 2 Detoxification

When the liver is sluggish, Phase 1 of the detoxification cycle may not be processing toxins at a normal and necessary speed. This causes toxins to accumulate in the bloodstream. If the hormone estrogen, for example, is not dismantled during Phase 1, the buildup can reach potentially harmful levels. Premenstrual tension can be an expression of this. Many factors can cause Phase 1 to become sluggish. As we age, our detoxification processes slow. Use of medications such as anti-ulcer drugs (cimetidine) and oral contraceptives; exposure to cadmium, lead, and mercury; and consumption of large amounts of sugar and hydrogenated fats hinder Phase 1 detoxification.

Substances that slow down Phase 1 detoxification, setting the stage for a toxic buildup, are called Phase 1 inhibitors. They affect the DNA of the liver cells, causing less detoxification enzymes to be produced. In addition to those mentioned previously, Phase 1 inhibitors include:

- Grapefruit

- Turmeric

- Capsicum (found in hot peppers)

- Cloves

- Drugs containing benzodiazepene such as anti-depressants and Valium

- Antihistamines

- Ketoconazole (used in antifungal medications)

- Toxins from bacteria in the intestines

A different type of detoxification problem develops if Phase 1 breaks down toxins at so fast a rate that Phase 2 cannot keep up. In this situation, the toxic intermediates produced during Phase 1 waiting to be washed out in Phase 2 flood the system. Many of these intermediate compounds—stuck in between Phase 1 and Phase 2—are more dangerous than the original toxin. This bottleneck can become a biochemical nightmare, damaging the liver, brain, and immune system.

Some of the substances that accelerate the breakdown of toxins in the liver by increasing the production of Phase 1 enzymes, without a concurrent increase in Phase 2 enzymes, are known carcinogens—pesticides, paint fumes, and cigarette smoke. Others are well known for their detrimental effects, such as alcohol and steroids. Even some otherwise harmless substances, such as limonene from lemons, increase Phase 1 detoxification. But unlike cigarette smoke, limonene does not create dangerous intermediate molecules. As you read the following list, keep in mind that it is not strictly a list of "bad" things, but of those things that increase the rate of Phase 1 detoxification, and that this becomes a problem *only* when Phase 2 can't keep up.

- Phenobarbital

- Steroids

- Sulfonamide medications

Pancreatitis and the Detoxification Bottleneck

Mainstream medicine generally does not favor bottleneck detoxification problems in diagnosis and treatment. Our clinical experience, however, has shown us that when treatment focuses on eliminating this problem, other disease conditions improve. For example, we believe that many cases of pancreatitis are caused by a bottleneck detoxification problem. The use of alcohol, cigarettes, and a body-abusing lifestyle creates this bottleneck, and the free radicals generated in this process cause inflammation in the pancreas.

We had a patient who had been in the hospital several times for acute pancreatitis. He was always alternating between a healthy lifestyle and use of alcohol and cigarettes. After every binge, he would end up in the hospital with pancreatitis. We put him on a detoxification program with great success. Patients with pancreatitis often report exposure to diesel fumes, solvents, and trichloroethylene. These toxins also seem to accentuate the susceptibility to alcohol-related pancreatitis.

The treatment of pancreatitis with detoxification medicine is not mentioned in medical literature. However, we believe there is ample evidence to make it a first-line treatment consideration.

- Foods in the cabbage family
- Charbroiled meats
- High-protein diets
- Citrus fruits
- Vitamin B_1

- Vitamin B$_3$

- Vitamin C

- Environmental toxins (exhaust fumes, paint fumes, dioxin, pesticides)

- Cigarette smoke

- Alcohol

- Endotoxins from intestinal bacteria in the bloodstream

Research has shown that specific foods and nutrients not only have a beneficial effect on detoxification capability but can also provide a safe and viable approach to treating a variety of immune disorders and toxicity syndromes.

Exposure to a toxin, when coupled with exposure to another substance that speeds up Phase 1, is especially dangerous. The combination of alcohol and acetaminophen provides a good example. It's not uncommon to drink heavily and later take acetaminophen for the headache that follows. The intermediate compound (from acetaminophen) is an extremely toxic substance called n-acetyl-p-benzoquinoneimine (NAPQI). Under normal conditions, NAPQI

Case History

Joanie was a forty-eight-year-old female who had a history of hepatitis B, a disease of the liver. She had worked for many years in the graphic arts field and was regularly exposed to volatile organic solvents. She came to our clinic with symptoms of chronic fatigue. We did a comprehensive liver detoxification screening. The test clearly showed which pathways were out of balance. After recommending the correct nutrients, Joanie was on the road to repairing her damaged liver function and rebuilding her health.

is removed quickly during Phase 2, but alcohol intake forces more NAPQI into the liver than Phase 2 can handle.

If two or more detoxification accelerants are combined, they can interact, with serious consequences. An individual on a prescription medication who smokes, for example, actually needs higher dosages of the medication because smoking causes the medication to be broken down faster than it normally would be during Phase 1. If Phase 2 can't handle the extra burden, a detoxification bottleneck results. We predict that in the future, medical specialists will check detoxification capabilities in order to give more accurate drug prescriptions.

Problems in Phase 1 and Phase 2 liver detoxification are so prevalent and have such a major impact on health that we believe it's a good idea for everyone to have liver detoxification tests as part of a standard medical workup. This lab test, described in chapter 7, can identify problems localized in the different detoxification pathways. If you suffer from chronic liver and gallbladder problems, you're probably a candidate for this test. Abnormal results, of course, will require ruling out a liver disease before going ahead with detoxification therapy. Assessing detoxification function makes it possible to diagnose a problem before symptoms actually appear. Tests that measure Phase 1 and Phase 2 enzymes take much of the guesswork out of estimating the severity of liver detoxification dysfunction and can to some extent indicate whether a person is at special risk for cancer, neurological disease, chemical and drug sensitivity, and immune problems.

Diet and Detoxification: Feeding Phase 1 and 2

You can take steps to keep your liver detoxification system running smoothly. Diet has a strong effect on detoxification enzymes, and foods can help "regulate" or balance Phase 1 and Phase 2 activity. Eating foods that support the liver can reduce your susceptibility to damage from toxins and to conditions such as multiple chemical sensitivity syndrome, chronic fatigue syndrome, and cancer. Research has shown that specific foods and nutrients not only have a beneficial effect on detoxification capability but can also provide a safe and viable approach to treating a variety of immune disorders and toxicity syndromes.

Essential fatty acids are vital for Phase 1 detoxification, and the standard American diet does not provide an adequate supply of these vital nutrients. Essential fatty acid intake in the form of cold-water fish and flaxseed oils have a demonstrated ability to heighten detoxification. Other sources of essential fatty acids include edible oils, such as those made from sunflower seeds, walnuts, and sesame seeds; wheat germ; and supplements of black currant seed, borage, or evening primrose oil.

Eating fresh fruits and vegetables daily is a good way to continually replenish your body's store of glutathione, necessary for one of Phase 2's pathways. High-quality protein nourishes both the amino acid and the sulfation pathways. Vegetable sources of sulfur for the sulfation pathways include radishes, turnips, onions, celery, horseradish, string beans, watercress, kale, and soybeans. Eggs, fish, and meat are also excellent sulfur sources.

Cabbage, brussels sprouts, broccoli, citrus fruits, and lemon peel oils support Phase 2 activity. Studies have shown dramatic results from consuming broccoli sprout extract, which inhibits the activity of Phase 1 enzymes and simultaneously enhances the Phase 2 glutathione pathway. Broccoli sprout extracts are especially beneficial for people who have frequent or high-level exposure to pesticides, exhaust fumes, paint fumes, cigarette smoke, or alcohol. Anyone who is exposed to known carcinogens will benefit from broccoli sprout extract.

Adding herbs, spices, and foods that support Phase 1 and Phase 2 enhances detoxification. A detoxification diet of rice, fruits, and vegetables, with the addition of special vitamins and herbs, supports Phase 1 and Phase 2 detoxification enzyme systems.

Foods to Support Liver Detoxification

- Cabbage family
- Cold-water fish
- Flaxseed oil
- Fruits (fresh)
- Garlic
- Nuts and seeds
- Onions
- Safflower oil
- Sesame seed oil
- Sunflower seed oil
- Vegetables (fresh)
- Walnut oil
- Wheat germ and wheat germ oil

Nutritional Supplements to Support Liver Detoxification

- Bioflavonoids
- Black currant seed oil
- Borage oil
- Carotenes
- Coenzyme Q_{10}
- Copper
- Evening primrose oil
- Folic acid
- Iron
- Lecithin
- Magnesium
- Manganese
- N-acetyl-cysteine
- Niacin
- Riboflavin
- Selenium
- Silymarin (milk thistle)
- Trace minerals
- Vitamin A
- Vitamin B_6 (pyridoxine)
- Vitamin B_{12}
- Vitamin C (ascorbic acid)
- Vitamin D
- Vitamin E
- Vitamin K
- Zinc

The Gallbladder, Bile, and Gallstones

The gallbladder is the end of the detoxification road that begins in the liver. Bile is the fluid into which the liver excretes its toxins. (The other routes of elimination are the sweat glands and the kidneys.) After bile is produced in the liver, it runs into the gallbladder and eventually into the intestinal tract. We have found that in many cases people with liver problems also have gallbladder problems, and vice versa.

Bile is made in the liver from cholesterol, bilirubin, and lecithin and is then secreted into the gallbladder. While in the gallbladder, bile is concentrated by a reabsorption of the liquids into the circulatory system. A proper ratio of bile components is necessary for it to remain in solution. Abnormal ratios promote the formation of cholesterol crystals or stones in the gallbladder. During a meal, bile is secreted by the gallbladder into the intestines to promote the digestion and breakdown of oils and fats. After the intestines absorb them, these bile-digested fats are used in the body to build cells, hormones, and prostaglandins (a group of chemicals that act like hormones).

When constipation occurs, bacteria in the intestines split the toxins that are bound up in the bile, in turn causing reabsorption of these already detoxified poisons. A diet high in vegetables will prevent constipation. Beta-glucuronidase is an intestinal bacterial enzyme that releases compounds for reabsorption. To prevent this reabsorption of toxins, an adequate supply of calcium d-glucarate, a natural ingredient in vegetables that inhibits beta-glucuronidase activity, is necessary. Charcoal will also bind up the bile and prevent toxins from being reabsorbed into the bloodstream.

Gallstones—a common complaint in North America—easily disrupt the flow of bile. They are found in sixteen to twenty million Americans and are twice as common for women as men. Usually the stones are a mixture of cholesterol, calcium, bilirubin, and lecithin. Occasionally, however, the gallbladder also forms a stone consisting mainly of calcium with a little bit of cholesterol. If you have gallstones, observe the following instructions:

1. Take lecithin daily. Cholesterol stones are caused when your liver excretes more cholesterol into the gallbladder than it does lecithin and bile acids. The cholesterol tends to "supersaturate" and form stones. A daily supplement of 500 mg of lecithin with meals keeps the bile flowing smoothly.

2. Limit dietary sugar. Sugar intake correlates with gallstone formation, suggesting that sugar stimulates cholesterol synthesis.

3. Take 5 g of soluble fiber (pectin in fruits, beans, or oat bran) daily with meals.

4. Eat a low-fat diet to prevent obesity.

5. Eat small meals to ensure proper digestive capacity.

6. Avoid food allergens, which are notorious for provoking acute attacks of gallbladder inflammation. Eggs are considered the worst offender.

7. Take 500 mg of bile acids with every meal; this is usually 50 percent effective in reducing the size of the cholesterol variety of gallstones.

8. Take supplements of the amino acids methionine and taurine. Because women's bodies make less taurine than men's, this might be the clue to their twofold increased risk for gallstones. The dose is 1 g of each, between meals, twice daily.

9. Take dandelion root *(Taraxacum officinalis)* extract. It's a superb cholegogue (releases stored bile), gentle in action, and safe to use. The dose of the solid extract is 1 teaspoon, 3 times a day. The solid extract is hard to find in the store, but the next best thing is to use the powdered root. The dose is 8 g as a tea, 3 times a day.

Detoxification and You

Human beings are not created biochemically alike. Everyone has a liver and a gallbladder; all livers and gallbladders are designed to do the same work; but not all livers and gallbladders work the same. Some of us are genetic warriors—naturally equipped to stay up all night, drink alcohol, eat whatever we like, smoke, and work brutal hours under tremendous stress—and even so die peacefully in our sleep at the age of ninety-five. But for others, not born with a hardy, resilient constitution, such a lifestyle is a prescription for poor health and an early death. Despite the fact that advertisements for everything from painkillers to breakfast cereals create the impression that what's good for one is good for all, there is really a large range of variability in how we function metabolically and what we need.

Genetic biocapabilities determine, to a large extent, our ability to handle the onslaught of environmental toxins.

Each of us faces the physical, mental, and emotional stresses of life equipped with a unique molecular system characterized by its own inherent weaknesses and strengths. These genetic biocapabilities determine, to a large extent, our ability to handle the onslaught of environmental toxins. For example, much of the variability in the activity of both the glutathione and the sulfation pathways is inherited. Your inborn capacity to manage toxins creates the climate in which either health or disease will flourish. A family history of estrogen-related breast cancer, smoking-induced lung cancer, and other types of cancer can be related to inherited weaknesses of detoxification capability.

These genetic differences are a result of the wide variance in how detoxifying enzymes in the liver express themselves. The term to describe this is *metabolic polymorphism*. This means that there is a variety *(poly)* of forms *(morphism)* that humans have in detoxifying their environment *(metabolic)*.

In the book titled *Genome*, authors Jerry E. Bishop and Michael Waldholtz propose that genetic susceptibility factors should be the major focus of medicine in the future. This, they suggest, would make it possible to modify the environment appropriately to protect individuals against diseases related to genetic polymorphism. Yet hereditary variations in the biochemical breakdown and transformation of toxins is still one of the most undervalued and underutilized areas of prevention and treatment.

Medical doctors could be individualizing health care plans and minimizing risks using laboratory tests (described in chapter 7) to assess detoxification functions. This screening process would identify those individuals who have very strong detoxification abilities as well as those who require special help to discourage the onset of disease. Not taking genetics and detoxification abilities into consideration sets the stage for illnesses that are preventable.

It is possible to minimize the impact of our biological weak links. The "Achilles' heel" that's encoded in our DNA makes each of us more susceptible to certain stressors can be countered by our daily lifestyle choices and compensated for with nutritional medicine and detoxification support. Naturopathic doctors have many ways to stimulate the liver, for example, using herbs, special diets, physiotherapy, and homeopathic medicines. Treatment of gallbladder disease frequently includes the same herbal medicines that are used for liver detoxification problems. If you have an inherited weakness in these organs, the EcoTox program will help. It is designed to stimulate the liver and gallbladder as well as the proper digestion of foods and nutrients necessary for their activity. In the following chapter, you'll learn more about the sources of toxins that place such a heavy burden on the liver and the toll they take on your health.

CHAPTER 6

We're In-Toxin-Cated

Living "Under the Influence" of Toxins

- Toxins in Unexpected Places
- Air Pollution
- Water
- Food
- Pesticides and Herbicides
- Heavy Metals

Being in-toxin-cated is like being intoxicated—both conditions seriously impair your ability to function normally and put you at risk. The big difference is that you know the source of your inebriation, and, unless you're a full-blown alcoholic, you can choose whether or not to go on a drinking binge. We can decide not to smoke or use recreational drugs, both major causes of in-toxin-cation, or choose to avoid working with hazardous industrial or agricultural chemicals. But many things that poison our system and put us "under the influence" are parts of the food we eat, the air we breathe, the water we drink, and products of the polluted internal environment of our own malfunctioning bodies. With a few exceptions, we don't see, smell, or taste most of the toxic substances we are exposed to every day. No matter how conscientious you are, it is becoming more and more difficult to completely control your exposure to toxins.

This chapter is about the causes and sources of our in-toxin-cation. Armed with this information, each of us is better equipped to limit our exposure and protect ourselves. Once you understand that toxins are ever present and all around, accumulating slowly in your body like water from a leaky faucet dripping into a bucket, you'll also realize why detoxification is so important. If you don't empty the bucket, eventually it will overflow: That toxic overflow is the beginning of disease and disability. When your detoxification system is overworked, your exposure to environmental poisons becomes even more problematic, and toxins take an increasingly greater toll on your health. Detoxification is the way to empty your bucket.

Toxins in Unexpected Places

When you know a material is hazardous to your health, you do your best to avoid it or take precautions to safeguard yourself. Unfortunately, the toxicity of many materials is not always obvious. Some substances used in common household and office products are a source of toxins and pose a potential health hazard to chemically sensitive individuals and to those with impaired or overwhelmed detoxification capabilities. If you feel that you or members of your family are at risk, try to replace the following items whenever possible with toxin-free alternatives.

Bedding. Foam rubber pillows and mattresses release chemicals. Cotton mattresses are laced with pesticides and fire retardants that can cause toxicity in the nervous system.

Cleaning materials. The chemicals commonly found in cleaning compounds are phenols, formaldehyde, toluenes, xylene, methylene chloride, and butane—all of which are dangerous to the immune and nervous systems.

Soft vinyl floors. Dangerous chemicals found in floors include butanols, trichloroethylene, toluene, benzene, xylene, phenols, hexanes, and styrene. Exposure to benzene can cause infertility, aplastic anemia (a problem localized in the bone marrow), and white blood cell chromosome damage, and it is also linked to leukemia. The effects of being exposed to a wide variety of chemicals for those with sensitive immune systems (for example, babies) are still unknown. Hard vinyl might be a better choice as it is safer and more inert.

Office supplies. Copy machines and correction fluid emit trichloroethylene (TCE), which is also used in dry cleaning products, rug shampoos, floor polishes, and old anesthetics. This substance has been known to cause confusion, inability to concentrate, fatigue, poor reaction time, peripheral neuropathy, poor coordination, headache, and muscle cramps.

Cosmetics. Some cosmetics contain nitrosamines, which have been found to cause cancer. Beauty shops pose a high risk of exposure. Black hair dye contains mutagenic chemicals, which can cause changes in the DNA code (a precursor of cancer), and, if used for more than twenty years, it poses a four times greater risk for contracting non-Hodgkin's lymphoma and multiple myeloma (a type of leukemia).

Job-Related Toxins. Table 6.1 lists some common chemical compounds, their occupational source, and the type of cancer to which they may be linked.

Table 6.1. *Industrial and Occupational Hazards*

Compound	Occupational Source	Cancer
Aromatic amines	Manufacturing chemicals, coal, gas, rubber	Bladder
Arsenic	Pesticide manufacture, mining substances	Skin, lung
Asbestos	Asbestos manufacture, applications (e.g., car brakes)	Lung, abdomen
Benzene	Glues, varnish	Leukemia
Bischloro-methylether	Certain types of resins	Lung
Cadmium	Refining	Prostate
Chrome ores	Manufacturing	Lung
Coal products	Chimney sweeping	Scrotum
Mustard gas	Manufacturing	Lung, larynx
Nickel ores	Refining	Lung, sinuses
Polycyclic hydrocarbons	Combustion of coal and mineral oils	Skin, lung
Shale oil	Tar and pitch exposure	Skin
Vinyl chloride	Leather and shoe industry	Sinuses
Vinyl chloride	Polyvinyl chloride manufacture	Liver
Vinyl chloride	Rubber processing	Lung
Wood dust	Hardwood furniture	Sinuses

SOURCE: Adapted from *Wellness Medicine* by Robert Anderson (Lynwood, WA: American Health Press, 1987).

Air Pollution

During the air pollution alerts in London in 1952, four thousand people died and tens of thousands became ill. Our air—and the pollution it carries—might be one of the greatest health risks. For example, it was found that people who smoke in polluted cities have a fourfold risk of developing emphysema. The air pollution measured by government agencies is caused mainly by industry and automobiles. The damage of this pollution is clearly demonstrated by examining its effects on human populations. Asthma rates have risen dramatically over the past few decades, especially among those who are often more immunologically vulnerable: the young and old. The rise in the incidence of asthma parallels the rise in automobile emissions. Increases in the number of emergency room visits for acute asthma attacks correlate with the higher levels of airborne particles as reported in air pollution statistics.

Air in the Home and Office

The baby-boomer generation is the first to grow up exposed on a regular basis to plastics and petroleum-based chemicals, which include new compounds the immune and detoxification systems had not seen fifty years ago. The industries that created such substances likely didn't conceive of the devastating effect on human health that these substances can create.

The building industry produces invisible and unmeasured air pollution. The highest concentrations of construction chemicals can be found in newly constructed offices, shopping malls, schools, and hospitals. Carpets, plywood, cabinets, and particleboard contain phenols, acetone, toluene, xylene, benzene, polystyrene, ethanol, styrenes, and formaldehyde. The use of "tight buildings" (those in which windows can't be opened and that have closed ventilation systems that constantly recirculate the air) has concentrated our exposure to formaldehyde and other "gassed" toxins from building materials. Carpet glues, in addition to many of the chemicals that are emitted from new carpets, are very toxic. Construction practices depend heavily on wood, and due to dwindling supplies, consumers are encouraged to use materials such as particleboard, which is made with glues and chemicals that contain formaldehyde, which can cause headache and fatigue. In 1982, ureaformaldehyde insulation became notorious for causing headaches, eye irritation, nausea, respiratory ailments, depression, dizziness, and fatigue.

Unfortunately, the risks of chemical exposure are often not well communicated in the workplace. People usually find out about chemical sensitivity after they have already become sick. Children in the Los Angeles area who develop brain tumors are three times as likely to have parents who have repeated on-the-job contact with chemicals, solvents, and paints either through physical contact or by inhaling the fumes. These workers are usually employed in chemical, aircraft, and industrial occupations. Researchers now recognize that some childhood cancers are related to carcinogen exposure during gestation. It's likely that the children's brain tumors are precipitated by their exposure to toxins while still in the womb.

It's also been noted that people who live around refineries also have a higher incidence of lung cancer than those who do not.

Water

The water rushing out of the faucet may look crystal clear, but it isn't. Drinking water has been found to be a toxic chemical soup. In 1993, the Environmental Protection Agency found 819 cities with lead in their water supplies that exceeded acceptable levels. Congressionally sponsored investigations by the GAO (General Accounting Office), as well as those performed by environmental watchdog groups, have repeatedly uncovered violations of clean water standards in systems around the country.

According to the Kellogg Report issued by the Institute of Health Policy and Practice of the Bard College Center, the growth of industry since the beginning of the twentieth century has been responsible for the introduction of new, complex, and sometimes lethal pollutants into our nation's water systems. The report, which examines the relationship between the health of the American people and nutrition, environment, and lifestyle, highlights the fact that municipal treatment plants neither detect nor detoxify the water supply of the majority of chemical pollutants, leaving the stuff that flows out of our taps "as badly tainted with chemicals as they were with bacteria before chlorination."

Contact your local, county, or state water agency to obtain the test results for your own local water. You can reduce your exposure to these chemicals by buying a home water filtration system or by drinking only purified water. The three types of systems available are solid block carbon filters, reverse osmosis, and distillation. Some offer a combination of methods. Good systems are not cheap, but ensuring access to clean water is a good health investment. There are many systems on the market—decide what you can afford, do your research, and purchase one from a reputable dealer. It would be a good idea to choose systems certified by the NSF (National Sanitation Foundation).

Food

Your diet has a powerful impact on your health; it's a leading source of toxins and a minor source of nutrients. It is a sad but true fact that much of our food supply is contaminated, and often what we eat lacks the essential vitamins, minerals, enzymes, fatty acids, and phytochemicals (plant-based nutrients) we require. Animals that end up on our dinner plates are fattened with drug-laced feed, and many of the fish we eat swim in polluted waters.

Fruits and vegetables are also likely sources of toxins. The ground in which our fruits and vegetables are grown is riddled with the chemicals of agricultural and industrial runoff. Fresh produce is harvested before it's ready, then sprayed with chemicals to force ripening. The grain used to make our bread, cake, and pasta is sprayed with noxious poisons designed to kill living organisms. There are 400 different pesticides that can legally be used in this country on food crops. Of the 268 million pounds of pesticides sprayed on California crops in 1980, 7.8 million pounds were found to be carcinogenic in test animals. In addition, large-scale farming practices, including the use of chemical fertilizers, deplete the soil of vital nutrients, which leads to the production of food that lacks the fundamental building blocks of life and the nutrients your body needs to protect itself from toxins.

With a few exceptions, we don't see, smell, or taste most of the toxic substances we are exposed to every day.

Packaged foods are laden with unnatural, unhealthy additives and preservatives; thousands are currently in use. Processing and refining further depletes the nutritional content of the foods we're consuming every day.

Toxicity from Food Reactions

Based on years of practice, nutritionally oriented clinicians of all types are convinced that food sensitivities and reactions to the toxins in some foods constitute the basis of most disease conditions. It's not very hard to grasp the concept that heavy metals, lethal herbicides and pesticides, chemical ad-

Case History

Allergic reactions to foods can cause problems in even the healthiest of people. Ed was a forty-year-old karate instructor and a generally healthy, active, and vital person. However, he suffered from some annoying health problems, including fatigue, headaches, and stomach and shoulder pain. We recognized his complaints were due to food allergies that had chronically irritated his intestinal tract. Though easily taken care of at this point, his condition eventually could have led to debilitating arthritis and bowel disease. We put him on a detoxification program and advised him to stay away from foods to which he showed sensitivity. Taking this approach will reduce his need for doctor visits and prescription medications in the future and allow him to feel healthier and happier in the present.

ditives, and air pollutants are poisonous. It is, however, more difficult both to understand and accept that if we're biologically intolerant of certain ingredients, even the most ordinary and delicious foods become toxic substances for our bodies; they irritate the intestinal tract, prompt the immune system to react, and stress our detoxification capabilities.

A complex biochemical interplay between what you eat and your intestinal environment contributes to food sensitivities and reactions. Genetic defects resulting in decreased production of necessary digestive enzymes, as well as an excess of gut toxins, repeated use of antibiotics that destroy helpful bacteria, intestinal permeability, and the presence of high levels of stress hormones all contribute to an individual's reactivity. Intolerances, or food allergies, can take many different forms of symptom manifestation. Reactions to food allergies can cause hives, asthma, nasal inflammation, nasal polyps, headaches, upper abdominal pain, and mood changes. Abdominal pain, vomiting, diarrhea, and poor growth are common symptoms in children with food allergies. Chronic pediatric ear infections have also been linked with food allergies.

Chocolate, coffee, tea, cola, bananas, tomatoes, avocados, cheese, pineapples, and wine contain vasoactive amines (neurotransmitters) that cause headaches, flushing, and nervousness in sensitive individuals. Food additives, such as dyes, have been implicated in aggravating the symptoms of hyperactivity in some children. Other common food additives that cause reactions are benzoates, acetylacetic acid, and tartrazine and other synthetic colors.

The most common foods associated with food sensitivities are wheat and other gluten-containing grains and cow's milk (including all products made with it). Many of our patients are surprised when we make strong recommendations to avoid these staples of the North American diet.

Eating allergenic foods is one of the main causes of intestinal permeability. If the intestinal membrane is highly permeable, food antigens, bacterial toxins, dietary peptides, and other toxic substances leak into the bloodstream. Identifying foods that prompt allergic reactions and sensitivities and eliminating them from the diet is an essential part of detoxification. As long as individuals continue to eat foods to which they react, healing cannot take place. Discovering which foods cause food allergy can be done using an elimination diet or can be diagnosed with a blood test. (See chapter 7 for more information.)

Rancid Oils

The molecular structure of plant-based oils is very fragile. Edible oils are sensitive to, and easily damaged by, oxygen, light, and heat. Foods that contain oils spoil quickly when exposed to air. Cooking, especially at very high heat, also damages oils, altering their molecular connection so that they become poisonous to the body. Rancid oils, made toxic by either oxygen or heat exposure, should not be consumed. They can be identified by their characteristic "bad" smell.

Some oils are more prone to rancidity than others. Olive oil, a monounsaturated fat, is the most stable oil and therefore a good choice for cooking. Oils sold on the supermarket shelves in clear glass or plastic bottles generally contain preservatives to keep them from spoiling. Oils sold in dark bottles or cans are preferable. Stale foods, deep-fried foods, old nuts, and packaged foods beyond their expiration dates should all be avoided because they could contain rancid oils.

Mold-Contaminated Foods

Although some molds are beneficial producers of anti-biotics, molds and fungi contain toxins that disturb the immune and detoxification systems. No one willingly eats bread, fruit, or vegetables with visible mold on them, but most of us are consuming moldy foods every day. Less-than-perfect fruit, much of it rotting and moldy, is typically used in the production of commercial juices. Nuts and grains, unless properly stored, readily grow a mold that produces a carcinogenic substance called aflatoxin. Peanuts and cottonseed oil are often contaminated with aflatoxin. Wheat flour and all the food products made with it are also especially vulnerable to aflatoxin contamination. Roasting nuts, seeds, and grains will kill the mold and inactivate the toxin.

Pesticides and Herbicides

The North American agricultural business depends on the use of pesticides and herbicides, which are infiltrating our bodies at an alarming rate. Organophosphates, which have an affinity for the nervous system, are among the most common. These substances, like so many other toxins, are especially harmful to the young, whose exposure to toxins may start before they are even born, and to the elderly. They increase nervous system activity and produce tremors and twitching, coordination problems, anxiety, hyperexcitablity, and a variety of learning disorders.

Our air—and the pollution it carries—might be one of the greatest health risks.

Many pesticides favored by the agriculture industry are carcinogenic and have contaminated our food and water supply. As Sandra Steingraber notes in *Living Downstream: An Ecologist Looks at Cancer and the Environment,* in Illinois alone there are an estimated 54 million pounds of synthetic pesticides applied to the farmlands. These substances often evaporate into the jet stream of our atmosphere and ultimately end up in groundwater aquifers, lakes, streams, and even in rain. We highly recommend this book for more detailed information about this very important subject.

Those pesticides that are not broken down by the detoxification system and eliminated get stored in fat tissues. One study found that in recent years the hexachlorobenzene content of fatty tissue had increased by 50 percent over previously sampled levels. Another study reported by the California Department of Consumer Affairs showed that individuals who had died of liver, brain, or neurological disease had higher pesticide residues in brain and fat tissue than people who had died of natural causes. The tendency of pesticides to accumulate in fatty tissues poses a special threat to dieters. When weight loss is not accompanied by a detoxification regimen, pesticides stored in fat are released.

People who work with pesticides and herbicides tend to have a higher incidence of cancer of the stomach, connective tissue, skin, brain, prostate, lymphatic system, and bone marrow. In a scientific study of a group of Saskatchewan farmers, adjusted for the use of pesticides, fertilizers, and farming practices, a direct correlation was found between herbicide use and non-Hodgkin's lymphoma (a cancer of the lymph glands). It was also found that the more spraying the farmers did, the more likely they were to die from the disease. Another study found an association between insecticide pest strips and childhood leukemia, childhood brain tumors, and childhood lymphomas. Yard pesticides have also been linked with soft-tissue sarcomas, and house insect pesticides were associated with adult lymphoma. A study involving dieldrin noted that cancer patients had higher levels of this pesticide in their bodies than noncancer patients.

The evidence tying pesticides to breast cancer is dramatic and impossible to ignore. Pesticides mimic estrogen (the body thinks they actually are estrogen and responds accordingly), and unnaturally high estrogen levels are known to promote cancer. An Israeli study conclusively related a drop in the incidence of breast cancer among Israeli women to a new law prohibiting the use of pesticides. The estrogenic effects of pesticides accelerate breast cancer and other hormone-sensitive cancers, an effect that is magnified when more than one type of pesticide is present or when combined with the consumption of large quantities of alcohol.

Heavy Metals

Most doctors don't include testing for the presence of heavy metals in their standard workup. Once these toxins are stored in tissues following initial exposure, they become harder to detect with tests that assess only blood levels. In our clinic, we screen all new patients for heavy metals using the highly accurate technique of hair analysis (a test described in chapter 7). This screen has found an incredible array of metals in the bodies of patients. People in some professions, such as dentists, welders, and plumbers, show especially high levels of heavy metals.

Most people have no idea that they have been exposed to these toxins. Mercury, aluminum, lead, and cadmium are the most commonly detected toxic metals. Heavy metals are particularly dangerous because they have a doubly toxic effect, damaging the inner workings of cells and at the same time impairing detoxification mechanisms, so that other toxins can cause even more damage than they otherwise would. Toxic metals, such as lead and cadmium, inhibit vital enzyme function (disrupting basic metabolic processes) and also increase free-radical production. Exposure to these metals can cause high blood pressure, artery disease, kidney disease, and neurological problems.

Toxic metals have two dangerous effects:

1. Heavy metals, being mutagens and carcinogens, modify the structure of DNA or interfere with the DNA-coding process, upsetting the communication between the DNA and the rest of the cell. Toxic metals also interfere with cell division. Cadmium causes the greatest disturbance in the normal process of cell division; in order, the next most harmful metals are mercury, cobalt, copper, nickel, and lead.

2. Heavy metals displace vital minerals such as zinc in enzymes and cell structures.

In any detoxification program, elimination of toxic metals is the first order of business. Any other treatment will be relatively ineffective unless these metals are removed from the body.

Aluminum

Aluminum is the most abundant mineral in the earth's crust. In the ground, in its natural chemical state, it is tightly bound in an inert, oxidized form so that it can't be absorbed by human tissues and get into the bloodstream.

Until a hundred years ago, aluminum toxicity was not a problem. However, since the late 1800s, when industrialists discovered a process for smelting aluminum, it has been a popular, inexpensive metal used to make cooking pots, cans, dishes, and wrapping for the food we eat. Processing and using aluminum in these products liberates it into our food and drink; it then migrates into the cells of our body. Because humans were not exposed to such high levels of aluminum earlier during our development, we did not acquire any detoxification mechanisms to deal with it. Instead, it is stored in our tissues, and when levels get high enough, it can cause a variety of health problems. The levels of aluminum inside our cells increase with age because we have no way to eliminate it from our bodies.

Aluminum damages cells by binding to phosphate molecules in the cell's DNA and RNA, altering the memory code. Imagine someone altering your secret code for your bank card without you knowing it. Suddenly, you have no access to your bank account. DNA is a cell's memory, and when the DNA protein transcription is disturbed, the cell can't get to the knowledge it needs to run various life processes. This leads to a sort of anarchy of cellular function. Aluminum damage can be compared to some instances of brain damage in which certain stored memories are lost and skills that took years of experience to accumulate are forgotten. This metal causes the cells to lose their memory in the same way; the cells that live a long time, such as neurons in the brain, seem to be the most affected.

If there are high levels of aluminum in the body, it can cause neuron changes in the brain, which may be associated with the neurofibrillary tangles found in Alzheimer's patients.

Such changes commonly cause diminished cognitive performance and neurological deficits, with loss of balance, memory loss, lack of coordination, and depression. In serious cases of aluminum toxicity, there will be seizures and dementia.

To limit exposure to aluminum, avoid all antiperspirants, antacids, and carbonated sodas that typically contain this heavy metal. Do not cook with aluminum pots or aluminum foil.

Lead

Lead exposure is causing a silent epidemic. This metal slowly accumulates in the body. Exposure can begin even before birth. With gradual exposure through food, water, or job-related contact, lead can destroy the nervous and cardiovascular systems. It shuts down detoxification enzymes and blocks enzymes in red blood cells that help carry oxygen throughout the body.

Lead has been poisoning human societies for thousands of years, though its damaging effects were not known until modern times. Early Greek civilizations used lead to make urns for storing wine because the sweet taste of the lead cut the acidic taste of the wine, and the Romans used it for connecting water pipes and making eating and drinking utensils. In more recent times, lead was an ingredient in gasoline and paint, until its dangers became well documented. Lead is also found in metal solders, ore smelters, lead water pipes and joints, and pottery glazes.

In ancient times, exposure to multiple toxins was unusual. Today, however, a huge variety of toxins are a part of everyday life. It's not uncommon to find levels of more than one heavy metal in individuals with multiple health problems. The most dangerous aspect of lead exposure is its interaction with other toxins. For example, lead has a combined effect with mercury that is very destructive. This is an example of toxic synergism, or toxins having an effect that is greater than the addition of the individual substances.

Lead also interacts with minerals in the body in an unhealthy way. The minerals iron and calcium increase lead absorption, and this absorbed lead tends to displace calcium in the bones. One study found that a pregnant mother's lead exposure could result in lead displacing the calcium in the fetus's bones. This can later manifest as dental cavities in young children. Zinc deficiency also increases lead absorption.

The most common foods associated with food sensitivities are wheat and other gluten-containing grains and cow's milk (including all products made with it).

The average daily intake of lead from water, cigarette smoke, air pollution, and food is 200 mcg. Fortunately, most of this lead is not absorbed and passes through the body. Unlike their inability to handle aluminum, our natural detoxification mechanisms are able to process the lead that is absorbed and excrete it in the urine, sweat, and feces. However, as exposure increases, these detoxification mechanisms are pushed beyond their capabilities.

Unfortunately, the signs and symptoms of lead contamination are common ailments that can be misdiagnosed as other disorders. They include constipation; poor appetite; abdominal pain; numbness in the fingers, toes, and lips; headache; tremors; a metallic taste in the mouth; joint pains; decreased nerve conduction; peripheral neuropathy (tingling and numbness in the hands and feet) and demyelination (loss of the protective sheath that surrounds the nerves, as in multiple sclerosis); attention deficit disorder in children; and dental cavities in children of mothers exposed to lead. The most common diseases caused by lead are atherosclerosis (hardening of the arteries), hypertension (high blood pressure), neurological diseases, anemia, kidney disease, learning disorders, and porphyrias (a disorder of hemoglobin metabolism).

Mercury

Mercury is the most toxic of the naturally occurring heavy metals. Amalgam fillings that contain mercury are considered by an increasingly large number of medical researchers to be a common cause of illness. Dental amalgams are the primary source of human exposure to mercury. A person with many amalgams could be absorbing up to 100 micrograms of mercury per day. Other significant sources are fish, fungicides used in agriculture, paints, lumber, coatings used in water-resistant fabrics, toys, and trace elements in fossil fuels.

Mercury toxicity was first documented in 1860 and described as "Mad Hatter disease" because felt-hat makers used mercury in their processing. The mercury contamination of Minimata Bay, Japan, in the mid-1950s caused more than three thousand documented cases of mercury poisoning. In 1972 methylmercury-contaminated seed grain in Iraq caused six thousand cases of poisoning and five hundred deaths. Today, South American villages and ecosystems are being poisoned by mercury as gold miners use it in their processing methods.

There is a wide range of symptoms to look for with low-level mercury toxicity: decreased sense of touch, hearing, vision, and taste; loss of appetite; numbness in the fingers, toes, and lips; excessive salivation; tremors; speech impairment; emotional disturbances; excitability; and nephrotic syndrome (damage to the kidneys that causes a failure to retain valuable proteins in the blood). Mercury toxicity is also implicated in stillbirths, spontaneous abortions, congenital malformations, decreased sperm production, chromosomal abnormalities, impotency, menstrual disturbances, and reproductive failures.

Dental amalgams are the primary source of human exposure to mercury.

There is no more destructive substance to human health than mercury. The organs most sensitive to damage by mercury are the intestines, kidneys, and nervous system. Mercury is a metabolic monkey wrench that gums up all the machinery inside a cell. Mercury is a mutagen (a substance that causes changes in cellular DNA) and a carcinogen that disturbs a cell's ability to divide or replicate. It also causes cellular damage by combining with sulfur molecules on membranes and in enzymes. This significantly disturbs energy production in the mitochondria. Mercury also disturbs immune function by altering the synthesis of DNA, and it upsets the blood-brain barrier.

The Danger of Amalgams Mercury has been used in silver dental fillings for years. Some dentists use a high-copper amalgam that releases five times the amount of mercury when compared to conventional low-copper amalgams. As amalgams deteriorate, mercury vapor and particles escape.

Chewing also releases mercury from amalgams. As mercury and other metals seep out of dental fillings into the highly absorptive area of the mouth, they leak into the bloodstream and are spread throughout the body. Studies have tracked mercury as it travels to many parts of the body, including the brain, kidney, jawbone, and gastrointestinal tract, and is stored in body tissues.

Once mercury is in the brain and kidneys, it begins to destroy the tissue. Because these changes are slow, symptoms related to brain function such as cognitive activity and changes in mood are hard to measure, but research has shown that these changes are nevertheless occurring. Studies also indicate that mercury alters the balance of intestinal bacteria and stimulates antibiotic resistance.

Patients with the following diagnoses should be screened for toxic levels of mercury:

- Lichen planus

- Cataracts

- Exercise-induced shortness of breath (anaphylaxis)

- Hormone dysfunction

- Inflammation of the kidneys (glomerulonephritis)

- Autoimmune disease

- Type IV immune reactions

- Multiple sclerosis

- Porphyrias

- Headaches

- Dementias

- Neurological diseases

- Kidney diseases

- Essential hypertension

In addition, people with the following chronic symptoms also should be screened for mercury toxicity:

- Loss of appetite
- Altered intestinal bacteria
- Depression
- Memory loss
- Swollen glands
- Nausea
- Insomnia
- Diarrhea
- Moodiness
- Gum disease
- Irritability
- Fatigue
- Headaches

If you have amalgam fillings, here are some valuable tips.

1. Avoid chewing gum. Mercury escapes up to twenty times faster from amalgams while chewing. Mercury levels as high as 87 micrograms per cubic meter of air have been measured after chewing gum.

2. Take regular supplements of acidophilus. See chapter 8 for more information.

3. If you are pregnant, do not have silver fillings placed in your teeth. Do not have those already in your mouth removed until after giving birth and ceasing to nurse.

4. If you have persistent neurological complaints that have not responded to standard treatment, have all dental

amalgams removed. There is a high positive correlation between the number and surfaces of dental amalgams and mercury levels of human brain tissue. Also, if you have any chronic immunological complaints, have all amalgams removed. Mercury fillings weaken the immune system.

5. If you are going to have dental amalgams removed, be sure it is done by a qualified practitioner of biological dentistry. A qualified dentist can be found by contacting the Foundation for Toxic Free Dentistry (P.O. Box 608010, Orlando, FL 32860-8010) or the American Academy of Biological Dentistry (P.O. Box 856, Carmel Valley, CA 93924). Excellent reading on the subject can be found in Sam Queen's *Chronic Mercury Toxicity* (Colorado Springs: Queen Health Communications, 1988).

Mercury doesn't stay in the blood except immediately after toxic exposure, but it is stored inside the cells in the body. Chronic low-level mercury is very hard to detect. Using human scalp hair samples, it's possible to detect mercury in the body as a result of amalgams and/or industrial, environmental, or dietary exposure. Another way to test for mercury is to use the saliva. By collecting a sample of saliva, it's possible to measure accurate levels of mercury release and a total mercury intake from amalgams.

Now that you are aware of what causes in-toxin-cation, you need to know about the cutting-edge technology that makes it possible to determine, when necessary, exactly what toxins are poisoning your body and burdening your mechanisms of detoxification. The next chapter describes the tests currently available.

CHAPTER 7

Laboratory Testing

Early Warnings

- **Regular Chemistry Screening Tests**
- **Acid/Base pH Testing**
- **A "New" Approach to Lab Testing**
- **Testing for Heavy Metals**
- **Functional Liver Detoxification Profile**
- **Oxidative Stress Testing**
- **Intestinal Permeability Testing**

- **Comprehensive Digestive Stool Analysis (CDSA) and Parasitology**
- **Food Allergy Testing**
- **Elimination Provocation Testing**
- **Organic Acid Analysis**
- **Amino Acid Analysis**
- **Vitamin and Mineral Assay**
- **Hormone Level Analysis**
- **Essential Fatty Acid Analysis**

The EcoTox program provides you with an effective treatment plan you can implement yourself. Laboratory tests are available that can help you optimize and individualize your detoxification program. Although you can still follow the detoxification program without these tests, they can help you, as well as your health care provider, apply detoxification strategies with more confidence and accuracy. In this chapter, we review the types of lab tests that are used to detect specific toxicity syndromes and detoxification problems.

Lab tests can reveal the precise nature of poor organ function and identify which ones are suffering from imbalances that may be the underlying cause of disease. With diagnostic testing that finds weaknesses in the functional ability of organs, it's also possible to treat disease before it happens. If you're already sick, these tests can also find disorders in organ function that other conventional tests might miss.

You can order some of these tests yourself. Ask your doctor for information about how to order them. If he doesn't know of labs specializing in these tests, try consulting a doctor versed in naturopathic or detoxification medicine. Some of these tests you can perform at home. Others must be performed by a qualified health care professional. Working with a trained practitioner can give you a deeper insight into the exact nature of your condition. Using these tests before and after a detoxification regimen is a way to document improvement, showing clearly that detoxification therapy is a valid medical strategy. An excellent resource for clinical laboratory testing is Great Smokies Diagnostic Laboratory (800-522-4762). They offer all of the tests mentioned in this chapter and can provide a referral to a physician in your area.

Regular Chemistry Screening Tests

Ask your doctor to do a full blood chemistry screen and then give you the results. Using the following information, try to make your own interpretation of the blood sample.

SGOT (serum glutamic-oxaloacetic transaminase), also called AST (aspartate aminotransferase) and SGPT (serum glutamic pyru-

vic transaminase), also called ALT (alanine aminotransferase). These liver enzymes are markers of cell damage in the liver and are a crude measurement for liver function. Look for elevated levels. Liver enzymes should always be on the low side. The normal range is from 0 to 40 IU/L, but I like to see the values under 30 IU/L. Niacin, vitamin A, alcohol, liver disease, and cancer metastases are factors that increase levels of SGOT and SGPT.

Bilirubin. Bilirubin is a by-product of hemoglobin metabolism in the body, the molecule that carries oxygen in the red blood cells. When the liver is sick, it loses the ability to process bilirubin, which backs up and can cause a yellow color in the eyes and skin. High bilirubin levels are seen in liver damage (hepatitis and infectious mononucleosis), in biliary duct obstructions (tumors and stones), and in hemolytic disease as well as prolonged fasting.

Calcium. The ideal calcium level is 10 mg%. Causes of elevated calcium include excess alcohol, sugar, coffee, vitamins A and D, hyperparathyroidism, cancerous tumors, osteoporosis, and drug therapy (thiazide diuretics, estrogens, and hyperthyroidism). Causes of decreased calcium include hypoparathyroidism, anticonvulsant drug therapy, calcium malabsorption, and chronic kidney disease.

Phosphorus. Ideal phosphorus levels are at 4 mg%. We have observed that low phosphorus levels are caused by inflammation and a poor diet. Chances of elevated phosphorus levels are increased by letting blood sit too long after it has been drawn. Other causes are hypoparathyroidism, vitamin D overdose, bone problems (Paget's disease and healing fractures), Addison's disease, magnesium deficiency, and diet (excessive ingestion of refined foods and drinks high in phosphoric acid, like soda pop).

Uric Acid. The most common cause of high uric levels in the blood is eating too much meat and drinking too much alcohol. These high levels of uric acid deposit crystals in the joints, causing the symptoms of gout. Uric acid levels in the blood are also increased by niacin, a high-protein diet, fish, wine, and fasting. Fasting increases these amounts because uric acid crystals are broken down during fasting, which may cause fasting-induced gout. One quart of cherry juice per day will decrease uric acid levels. Older men with cardiovascular disease are at risk for elevated uric acid levels due to the consumption of a high-meat diet and the use of hypertensive medication. Patients with lead poisoning and those who use weight-loss diets are also at risk of elevated uric acid levels. The normal range is from 3 to 7.6 mg/dl but an ideal range is under 6.2mg/dl.

BUN (blood urea nitrogen). Dietary protein increases blood urea nitrogen levels by 10 to 20 mg/dl. A vegan diet (no meat, eggs, or dairy products) decreases these levels and benefits the kidneys. Nephrotic syndrome (a type of kidney disease) produces high BUN levels, and it is hard to bring these values down. Ideal ranges are from 10 to 18 mg/dl. When the range is above 20 mg/dl, it indicates the beginning of kidney disease. From 50 to 150 mg/dl, it indicates serious kidney disease and from 150 to 250 mg/dl, there is definite severe impaired glomerular function. In chronic kidney disease, doctors usually use the BUN level as a better indicator for uremia than creatinine levels.

Creatinine. Creatinine is a test of kidney health. Conditions that can exhibit an increase in creatinine are a high-meat diet, muscle destruction from excessive exercise, kidney disorders, and gout. A fasting chemical screen is needed to test creatinine levels, as a diet containing meat will increase these levels. Creatinine levels are elevated by impaired kidney function. Protein should be reduced in the diet to bring down creatinine levels. Patients with elevated creatinine levels should be very cautious about receiving EDTA chelation therapy. A healthy range is from 0.8 to 1.1 mg/dl.

Cholesterol. Cholesterol levels are increased by coffee, sugar, vitamin D toxicity, and dietary saturated fat. Exercise and weight loss decrease cholesterol. Controversy over the optimum level places the range from 150 to 225. Indigenous people on hunter-gatherer diets typically have values lower than 180 mg/dl.

Fasting Blood Sugar. Glucose levels are increased by a diet high in refined carbohydrates, vitamin C, and niacin. Glucose levels greater than 90 mg/dl produce problems. Glucose levels are decreased by a diet low in refined carbohydrates, a diet high in soluble fiber (fruit/pectins and legumes), weight loss (improves insulin sensitivity), and exercise.

Ferritin. This easy-to-take test screens for low and high levels of iron stores in the body. Low iron stores predispose individuals to anemia, while high iron stores are a significant risk for atherosclerosis. The ideal range which is used by most athletes is 45 to 90 ug/l. Values of 18 to 45 are considered to be low. Under 18 ug/l are clinically significant. A serum ferritin which is too high generally is thought to be over 150 ug/l. In one study, men with serum ferritin greater than 200 ug/l had a 2.2-fold increased risk of acute myocardial infarction, compared to those with lower ferritin levels.

Acid/Base pH Testing

Checking the pH of your urine and saliva is a great way to determine how healthy the kidneys and liver are, the key organs of detoxification. In the Victoria clinic, I use a special machine that gives very accurate pH values, but you can also get excellent results by checking your pH at home. The Western diet and environmental toxins tend to decrease the pH of the body, making it more acidic. The result is an increased loss of calcium in the urine as the body tries to buffer itself against this unfavorable environment. Factors that tend to decrease the pH of the body include inflammation, oxidative stress, milk, and meat. Factors that increase the pH include eggs, poultry, whey protein, fruits, and vegetables.

Use the following procedure to measure your salivary pH and urine pH:

1. Swallow several times before testing saliva pH.

2. Discharge some saliva into a spoon and touch the pH paper to the saliva. Compare to the color chart after 30 seconds. Test the urine in a similar way by obtaining a specimen in a clean jar and dipping the pH strip into the urine.

pH Chart

	Saliva	Urine
Ideal	7.0–7.5	7.0–7.5
Margina	6.5	6.0–6.5
Risk for acidemia	<6.0	<5.5
Acidemia	<5.5	<4.5
Critical pH	<5.5	
High risk of alkalemia	>8.0	>8.0

Measure your saliva and urine before, during, and after your week of detoxification. Be pleased if you see a change in the pH in the correct range, especially if a chronic problem like arthritis improves at the same time.

A "New" Approach to Lab Testing

Pioneering labs in the rapidly evolving area of nutritional biochemical testing have developed many of the tests discussed in this chapter. These labs are found throughout North America, but their tests are not always integrated into conventional medical care, so your doctor might be unfamiliar with some of them. Although the tests described in this chapter have been well researched and are often covered by medical insurance and Medicare, they're still fairly new, and conventional medicine can take decades to integrate new science. If you can't order a certain test for yourself, either ask your doctor to order it or find a physician who knows about detoxification or naturopathic medicine. And remember that if you receive medical coverage through an HMO, you might have to pay for these tests out-of-pocket.

Most of the laboratories have staff members who are trained to discuss results with physicians and teach them how to use the principles of detoxification and functional medicine. We strongly recommend that your doctor call the lab for help interpreting the results.

With diagnostic testing that finds weaknesses in the functional ability of organs, it's also possible to treat disease before it happens.

Some labs are beginning to market tests to the public, allowing consumers to order and pay for lab tests that they think are important. For example, Great Smokies Diagnostic Laboratory is marketing hair mineral analysis and salivary hormone testing kits. You buy the kit from a local pharmacy or on the Internet. After the test is completed, the results give you a clearer picture of your health. This discussion will focus on many but not all of the common tests available.

Although we emphasize and encourage self-directed healing, sometimes the advice of a health care professional is necessary. The tests outlined in this chapter point to areas that might require exploration with someone who has more experience than you do. Because your biochemistry is complex and unique, figuring out what's wrong can be like looking for a needle in a haystack. It could take a combination of several different tests and a trained professional to interpret and synthesize the results in order to develop a personalized approach to detoxification treatment.

Finally, if you aren't feeling well, remember that there is a real reason. The EcoTox detoxification program is one way to address your health problems. If you don't get the results you hoped for after one week of detoxification, it doesn't mean the program has failed. Your problems may require a more specialized and intensive regimen, designed by a practitioner experienced in detoxification medicine. Remember, too, the benefits of internal cleansing continue in the weeks following your seven days on the EcoTox plan, especially for those who decide to modify their diet and lifestyle to lessen toxic exposure and accumulation. If you have not yet seen your regular doctor about your health problems and still feel unwell after following the detoxification program outlined in this book, it's also a good idea to explore some other, more conventional approaches.

Testing for Heavy Metals

Before considering any specific diagnostic protocols, such as an intestinal permeability test, we recommend that you begin by evaluating the burden of heavy metals on your body (see chapter 6). The most common heavy metals are cadmium, lead, mercury, aluminum, and nickel, and they are found in many of our patients who never suspected that they had any occupational exposure.

Minerals compose 4 percent of total body weight. The minerals our bodies carry in the largest supply are called macronutrients: calcium, potassium, sulfur, phosphorus, and sodium. Micronutrients are minerals that are found in smaller concentrations: magnesium, chromium, manganese, molybdenum, zinc, vanadium, selenium, and lithium. These minerals—macronutrients and micronutrients—are essential for good health. Without them, the body's immune and energy production systems can't work properly, and our ability to heal is impaired.

Unfortunately, these micro- and macronutrients are displaced by heavy metals, which mimic them. The body is tricked into using these dangerous toxins because it can't tell the difference between them and the real thing. For example, lead imitates calcium, and the body stores it in the bones. This contributes to a weakening of bone structure. As we discussed in the previous chapter, children whose mothers were exposed to lead while pregnant typically end up with weaker tooth structure and more dental cavities. Heavy metals also compete with certain minerals and upset many enzyme reactions inside the cells.

Step One: Hair Analysis

Hair analysis is a simple test for heavy metals that gives very reliable information. It provides a preliminary, inexpensive way to screen simultaneously for mineral imbalance and heavy metal toxicity. As hair develops inside the scalp, it's exposed to blood, lymph, and intracellular fluids. Thus, mineral levels in the hair follicles closely correlate with those in the body's tissues. Toxic metals concentrate in the hair hundreds of times faster than in the blood and can therefore provide an early warning tool for detecting toxic metals in the system.

In the test, a small amount of hair is cut from the nape of the neck and several other places. Only the inch and a half of hair closest to the head is used; this part of the hair follicle gives information about the past three months. People who have dyed, permed, or otherwise chemically treated hair must either wait to do this test until an inch and a half of untreated hair grows out or make sure that the lab knows exactly what product was used on the hair. For example, some dandruff shampoos have high selenium contents, which can throw off the results for hair selenium levels.

Hair analysis is an initial screening tool. If the results show imbalances, more thorough testing, done by a qualified health care professional, should follow.

Step Two: Urine Element Analysis

If your hair analysis shows toxic metal accumulation, the next step should be a urine element analysis administered by a doctor. This test can give diagnostic information about lead, cadmium, nickel, mercury, arsenic, beryllium, and aluminum in your body. This test is also used to monitor detoxification programs for metals by measuring how much of each metal is excreted in your urine.

In our clinic, a patient who needs to confirm a heavy metal toxicity is given an intravenous chelating drug that binds to these metals to help pull them out of the body. Urine is collected for twenty-four hours, shaken well, and measured, and then a portion is saved for analysis. The sample is picked up at one's home by an express shipping company and sent to the lab. Measurements of the various metals in the urine determine whether further treatment is necessary.

Functional Liver Detoxification Profile

As we have seen, the liver is an important metabolizer of toxic substances in the body. Most drugs, alcohol, pesticides, food additives, and nearly all foods pass through the liver's filtering system. A lab test called a functional liver detoxification profile makes it possible to determine how well your liver detoxification pathways are working. You test detoxification pathways by taking small amounts of "challenge" substances, such as acetaminophen, caffeine, and aspirin. Your urine is then measured for metabolites, the organic compounds produced by the breakdown of these substances in the liver.

Each pathway gives information about how you'll be affected by various drugs, foods, and xenobiotics, the term used for molecules foreign to biological organisms. For example, if an overload of Phase 1 detoxification enzymes shows up in the lab test, it indicates the potential for increased production of free radicals, leading to a greater risk of inflammatory diseases and cancer.

Another way to measure liver detoxification pathways is by measuring D-glucaric acid and mercapturic acid in the urine. D-glucaric acid is a general marker for Phase 1 detoxification pathways. By testing for it, we can detect the presence of xenobiotics, including pesticides, herbicides, fungicides, petrochemicals, and excessive alcohol intake. Mercapturic acid provides a measurement of glutathione conjugation, one of the Phase 2 detoxification pathways. People who can't tolerate caffeine, aspirin, or acetaminophen can use this test.

Oxidative Stress Testing

Oxidative stress testing measures the capacity of your body to withstand oxidative free-radical damage. For example, Phase 1 detoxification generates free radicals that are to be further broken down in Phase 2 and eventually washed out of the body. However, if left unchecked—as in the case of too rapid Phase 1 detoxification and/or blocked pathways in Phase 2—these by-products of poor detoxification can do great harm to your organs.

An oxidative stress test can help confirm damage from poor detoxification. Challenge substances—caffeine and aspirin—allow glutathione levels, lipid peroxides, and hydroxyl radical markers to be measured. Glutathione is one of the most active antioxidants, protecting us from free-radical damage because it regenerates vitamins E and C after they have been oxidized. Glutathione is also critical for maintaining red blood cells, and it enhances immune function. It is important for detoxification of heavy metals, certain medications, and bacterial toxins. The concentration of glutathione in the blood remains one of the most reliable indicators of total body glutathione, most of which is made in the liver and exported into the bloodstream.

Oxidative stress testing also screens for the presence of lipid peroxides and hydroxyl radicals, which have been linked to cell membrane damage from free radicals.

Intestinal Permeability Testing

As we discussed in chapter 4, most digestive activity and the absorption of nutrients into the bloodstream takes place in the intestines. If spread out flat, the intestines would cover an area the size of a tennis court. The intestinal walls are only about the thickness of an eyelid. To maintain the integrity of the intestinal membrane and repair any damage, the cells of this large yet fragile surface are completely replaced every three to five days. Stress, toxic overload, medications, excessive use of alcohol, altered gut ecology, smoking, poor diet, and illness inhibit this cellular repair and replacement activity. This leads to what is called "leaky gut syndrome" or intestinal permeability (see chapter 4).

Intestinal permeability testing can determine whether you have this condition, and it also can detect poor absorption of nutrients. The most common intestinal permeability test is the lactulose/mannitol test. Mannitol and lactulose are water-soluble sugar molecules that the body can't break down. Mannitol is a small molecule that is easily absorbed. You would expect to see high amounts of it in the urine. Lactulose is a large molecule that's poorly absorbed, so negligible amounts would be detected in the urine. A healthy person shows high mannitol and low lactulose levels. A person with increased intestinal permeability would have high levels of both mannitol and lactulose. Someone with poor absorption of nutrients would have low levels of both sugars in their urine.

Using these tests before and after a detoxification regimen is a way to document improvement, showing clearly that detoxification therapy is a valid medical strategy.

Any physician can order this test. You do part of it at home, first by collecting a random urine sample and then ingesting a mannitol/lactulose drink and collecting your urine for the next six hours. Both urine samples are sent to the lab for analysis. This test can be used for diagnosis and for monitoring how well your therapy is working.

Comprehensive Digestive Stool Analysis (CDSA) and Parasitology

The CDSA is an extremely important functional test. It allows us to see what is happening in your digestive system by looking at your stool. It shows:

- How well foods are being digested in the intestines
- How well you are eliminating toxic wastes through the stool
- How much good bacteria is present in your intestines
- The presence of unhealthy or pathogenic bacteria
- The presence of candida (yeast)
- The health of your colonic cells
- How well your immune system is handling the results of digestive tract activity

An imbalance in intestinal bacteria produces toxins that inflame and irritate tissues. If disease-causing bacteria or fungi are found, labs that do this comprehensive test culture can help determine which medications and natural substances would be the most effective treatment for you.

Intestinal parasite infestations are very common worldwide, even in North America. Many of us have grown up thinking that we are immune to these health problems, assuming that parasitic bowel infestations are a problem of third-world countries. However, more than 130 species of intestinal parasites have been found in North America.

Common symptoms of parasitic infestations include gas, bloating, diarrhea, fatigue, joint and muscle aches, itching, rashes, pain, sleep disturbances, unexplained fever, unexplained weight loss, and rectal bleeding. Labs that specialize

Parasite Infections

Although you don't necessarily need lab tests to get benefits from detoxification, such tests can be helpful to detect the cause of health problems that seem to resist conventional treatment. We recently worked with a man who had been diagnosed with irritable bowel syndrome. He had lost about twenty pounds and experienced bleeding with bowel movements, diarrhea, excessive fatigue, and stomach cramps. This had been going on for several months without improvement. His physician had done all the normal gastrointestinal testing, but found nothing unusual, and he prescribed anti-inflammatory medications to help heal the inflamed tissues. After several weeks, there was still no improvement.

He came to our clinic, and we performed a CDSA and tested for parasites and their eggs. We detected the presence of an amoeba as well as two bacteria that can cause diarrhea and cramping. This type of extensive intestinal workup has shown us that it is not uncommon for patients to have more than one bowel pathogen present at the same time. That's why in cases where there are chronic digestive difficulties we usually add a request for an ova and parasite examination on to the CDSA.

In cases such as this man's, we usually recommend papain enzyme therapy for the parasites (described in chapter 8). Bacterial infections of the bowel are treated with the EcoTox program with the addition of high doses of *Lactobacillus acidophilus* and *L. bifidus* (friendly probiotic intestinal bacteria). We also usually suggest supplementing with goldenseal: two capsules three times a day for a week. With appropriate treatment, this patient was feeling better in a matter of three weeks and realized he hadn't felt this well in years.

in parasitology often find parasites where other labs have failed. To be certain that parasites are not present, you would need to complete eight tests using the random-sample method that most labs rely on. Use of a laxative to provoke diarrhea enables labs to find parasites that lodge higher up in the colon. Some parasites live in the mucus and are most easily found by doing a rectal swab.

Under your physician's guidance, you can use a parasite testing kit at home as part of the CDSA by collecting one to four stool samples. The use of a rectal swab to examine the intestinal mucus for parasites must be done in the physician's office.

Food Allergy Testing

Food allergies and sensitivities play a role in an enormous variety of health problems. They can be inherited from one's parents, or they can be caused by intestinal infections, medications, or even stress. Once food allergies begin, the chronic inflammation they cause in the intestinal membranes and the leakage of food proteins into the bloodstream can cause severe health problems. A detoxification program is helpful, but to really heal it's necessary to determine which foods you are allergic or sensitive to and eliminate them from your diet for four to six months. During this time, your immune and digestive systems can recuperate; afterward, some of the foods might no longer bother you.

True food allergies affect only a small part of the population, but many people have food sensitivities (which can easily be confused with food allergies). True food allergies are mediated by a type of antibody called IgE. People tend to know about these allergies based on experience—you eat shrimp or strawberries and get hives, dairy products give you immediate diarrhea, and so on.

Case History

Sometimes you can't escape from contact with food allergens, especially if they're an integral part of your lifestyle. Detoxification can make your allergies easier to live with, however. Tom was the owner of a bakery, and ironically, he suffered from a severe wheat allergy. His reaction manifested mainly as a skin rash, which his doctor diagnosed as eczema. The symptoms accompanying the rash, involving itching and swelling, were terribly uncomfortable. Due to his occupation, he was continually exposed to wheat and his allergy was making life very difficult. We worked with Tom to set up a treatment plan of diet and nutritional supplements. Gradually his reactivity to wheat and the accompanying symptoms diminished. His allergy didn't disappear, because it was probably the result of a genetic inheritance, but he learned he could alter his allergic reactions through detoxification medicine.

Food sensitivities, on the other hand, are also known as delayed hypersensitivity reactions. Delayed reactions are exactly that: You eat something today, but tomorrow you have a migraine headache or wake up feeling groggy and tired or with bags under your eyes. These delayed reactions can underlie an enormous variety of symptoms and health conditions (for example, arthritis), many that you would never suspect were related to food allergies. Delayed reactions trigger antibodies called IgG. The IgG antibodies stimulate the immune system and create inflammation in many parts of the body.

Table 7.1 summarizes many food sensitivities and the symptoms that may indicate their presence.

Table 7.1. *Symptoms of Food and Environmental Sensitivity*

Note: The following symptoms can result from many different health conditions. Professional evaluation is necessary to uncover the source of these symptoms and to establish whether food sensitivities are involved.

Area Affected	Symptoms
Head	Chronic headaches, migraines, difficulty sleeping, dizziness
Mouth and throat	Coughing; sore throat; hoarseness; swelling and pain; gagging; frequently clearing throat; sores on gums, lips, and tongue
Eyes, ears, and nose	Runny or stuffy nose; postnasal drip; ringing in the ears; blurred vision; sinus problems; watery and itchy eyes; ear infections; hearing loss; sneezing attacks; hay fever; excessive mucus formation; dark circles under eyes; swollen, red, or sticky eyelids
Heart and lungs	Irregular heartbeat (palpitations, arrhythmia), asthma, rapid heartbeat, chest pain and congestion, bronchitis, shortness of breath, difficulty breathing
Gastrointestinal tract	Nausea and vomiting, constipation, diarrhea, irritable bowel syndrome, indigestion, bloating, passing gas, stomach pain, cramping, heartburn
Skin	Hives, skin rashes, psoriasis, eczema, dry skin, excessive sweating, acne, hair loss, irritation around eyes
Muscles and joints	General weakness, muscle/joint aches and pains, arthritis, swelling, stiffness

Table 7.1. *Symptoms of Food and Environmental Sensitivity (continued)*

Energy and activity	Fatigue, depression, mental dullness and memory lapses, difficulty getting your work done, apathy, hyperactivity, restlessness
Emotions and mind	Mood swings, anxiety, tension, fear, nervousness, anger, irritability, aggressive behavior, binge eating or drinking, food cravings, depression, confusion, poor comprehension, poor concentration, difficulty learning
Overall	Overweight, underweight, fluid retention, dizziness, insomnia, genital itch, frequent urination
Children*	Attention deficit disorder, behavior problems, learning problems, recurring ear infections

*These problems are often not recognized as being related to food sensitivities. Children with these problems will benefit from a food evaluation and environmental sensitivity testing.

SOURCE: *Digestive Wellness* by E. Lipski (New Canaan, CT: Keats Publishing, 1996).

IgE and IgG Blood Testing

Many physicians test only for IgE reactions. If only IgE tests are done, however, they'll miss some reactive foods. It's important to be tested for both IgE and IgG antibodies, so that you'll know to which foods you are truly allergic and to which ones you are sensitive. In this test, blood is drawn and sent to the lab. Your blood is put into little wells containing antibodies along with test foods. The lab technician measures the level of antibody reaction to each food.

Remember, too, the benefits of internal cleansing continue in the weeks following your seven days on the EcoTox plan, especially for those who decide to modify their diet and lifestyle to lessen toxic exposure and accumulation.

This test is sometimes a reflection of what you've been eating most recently. For example, if you know that dairy products and eggs bother you and you never eat them, they might show up negative on the test because you haven't eaten any for years. Because this test is measuring delayed hypersensitivity, occasionally a food that you've eaten but not noticed symptoms from shows up on the test results right away. An experienced clinician can help you decipher the test results.

Elimination Provocation Testing

A food allergy blood test is best used in conjunction with a test that you do at home: the elimination provocation test. This can easily be done in coordination with your detoxification program. Because you're eating a low-allergen diet during detoxification, all you have to do is slowly add one food every two to three days and gauge how you feel. Keep a detailed journal of what you eat and how you feel. Usually, after four to six days on the detoxification diet, many of your symptoms will have disappeared. By adding foods back slowly, it's easy to see which foods trigger symptoms. It takes persistence and perseverance, but this test is the most accurate way to discover your food sensitivities.

Wheat is a common irritant. If you're testing for wheat sensitivity, be sure to eat cracked wheat or bulgur wheat, preferably organically grown. Eat it two or three times for two days and see how you feel on the second and third day. If you notice symptoms, remove it from your diet for at least four days and retest. Sometimes you'll have to test a food three times before you're certain of your reaction. Maybe the wheat bothered you—or was it your hay fever? Or were you just run-down? Or was it the restaurant food you ate the day before? Be a supersleuth. It's worth the effort.

Organic Acid Analysis

Traditionally, organic acid analysis was used only to assess severe metabolic diseases in newborns. More recently, however, several other organic acid compounds have been found to be useful in detecting nutritional deficiencies and microbial imbalances. The most well known of these are homocysteine and methylmalonic acid.

Usually, after four to six days on the detoxification diet, many of your symptoms will have disappeared.

The Krebs (citric acid) cycle is a biochemical process for generating ATP (energy) inside the cells' mitochondria. Measuring organic acids can determine how well the Krebs cycle is working to generate ATP and where it is faltering. Specific nutrients and enzymes are known to facilitate each step of the Krebs cycle, which is why organic acid testing can be very useful for anyone who suffers from extremely low energy on a regular basis, such as patients with chronic fatigue syndrome. Certain toxicity syndromes are diagnosed using organic acid analysis.

Organic acid testing can also be useful for measuring how well your body is coping with toxins, for detecting fungal overgrowth and gut dysbiosis (bacterial overgrowth in the intestines), and for determining how well your body is able to utilize glucose and amino acids such as carnitine and tryptophan.

Your doctor must request the organic acid analysis, which is a urine-based test. However, your doctor might require assistance from a qualified biochemist consultant in interpreting organic acid analysis results.

Amino Acid Analysis

Amino acids are the building blocks of protein. We use protein for the maintenance and repair of cells and tissues and immune function. Because of genetic variations or environmental influences during their lifetimes, some people have difficulty absorbing specific amino acids from the foods they eat or manufacturing those considered nonessential (meaning the body makes them rather than obtains them from dietary sources). This produces a deficit of some amino acids and a surplus of others. Problems related to amino acid conversion can play a major role in athletic injuries, sleep disorders, thinking and memory problems, and attention deficit disorder in children.

In detoxification medicine, we measure amino acids in the urine and blood to see whether the proper balance exists to successfully run the detoxification machinery inside every cell. Amino acid testing can also determine whether your diet provides you with adequate protein and can help with diagnosis of vitamin and mineral deficiencies. Amino acid testing can provide relevant information about liver and kidney function, too.

Urine testing is the best method to use if problems have been chronic or lifelong. You collect samples of urine for twenty-four hours. Blood testing is used in cases in which the onset of symptoms is recent and to assess the current amino acid levels.

Vitamin and Mineral Assay

A conventional blood chemistry analysis gives blood levels of some vitamins and minerals, including sodium, potassium, calcium, phosphorus, and vitamin B_{12}. Unfortunately, for a complete nutritional picture, it's not sufficient to test serum levels of these nutrients. The most accurate method to check levels of some vitamins and minerals is to perform assays: Measurements of white blood cells, red blood cells, and enzymes necessary for the production of specific nutrients provide a much more accurate picture of what nutrient stores you have available in your body.

Many labs provide sophisticated analyses of vitamin and mineral status, showing whether levels of individual nutrients in the body are adequate. These tests are not very expensive and should be performed on anyone who has chronic illness. Vitamin and mineral status should also be carefully monitored throughout the duration of chelation therapy. Chelation drugs pull not only toxic metals from the body, but healthful nutrients as well. Monitoring nutrient levels helps you and your health care practitioner develop a plan for your supplementation program.

Hormone Level Analysis

Hormones deliver messages to cells about metabolism. When our hormones are in balance, we feel terrific. When they're out of balance, we can feel exhausted and/or depressed, have poor immune function and/or sexual problems, and get fat even though we don't eat too much. Poor liver detoxification can alter the healthy balance of hormones in our bloodstream because it's up to the liver to break down these molecules. Poor liver performance slows hormone breakdown rates.

There are two forms of hormones: bound and free. Bound hormones are not active until they are altered. Free hormones can be accurately measured in the saliva. Free hormones found in saliva easily pass through cell membranes, whereas bound hormones in the blood cannot. Conventional blood hormone testing groups together all free and bound hormones. Assessment of free salivary hormones gives a more accurate picture of what's really going on.

For example, a typical saliva hormone test screens for two adrenal hormones, cortisol and DHEA, and checks saliva levels four times daily. The results of these tests correlate with the actual levels of the hormones in your bloodstream. This can be very helpful in determining whether supplementation with DHEA is indicated. Low levels of DHEA have been found in people with chronic fatigue syndrome, lupus, arthritis, insomnia, high blood pressure, Alzheimer's disease, cancer, heart disease, and nearly all diseases associated with aging.

Men's and women's hormone panels are useful tools for evaluating sexual dysfunction; fertility problems; menstrual, perimenopausal, and menopausal problems; and prostate and impotency problems in men. Imbalanced sexual hormones can also cause significant changes in mood and behavior. People with insomnia and seizure disorders might want to test their melatonin levels.

Some of these hormone tests are available directly through pharmacies without the involvement of your physician. Great Smokies Diagnostic Laboratory has recently begun to market salivary hormone testing directly to the public through pharmacies and on the Internet. Their Web site is www.gsdl.com.

Essential Fatty Acid Analysis

We hear a lot about the health benefits of restricting fat intake. At the same time, however, many of us are fatty-acid deficient. Each day, we need about an ounce of essential fatty acids from our diet. These fats are essential to the health of cell membranes, brain function, nervous system, reproductive system, growth in children, and cardiovascular function. We eat enough fat—more than enough—but often not the right kind. Generally, our diets are high in trans fatty acids (harmful to our health) and omega-6 fatty acids and deficient in omega-3 fatty acids. The two types of fatty acids need to be present in the correct proportions: We need a 4:1 ratio of omega-6 fatty acids to the omega-3 fats.

A blood test for essential fatty acids can tell you whether you have deficiencies or excesses of omega-3 and omega-6 fatty acids, measure your level of trans fatty acids, and determine whether you have adequate amounts of GLA (gamma linolenic acid), EPA (eicosopentanoic acid), and DHA (docohexanoic acid).

Chronic toxicity syndromes can be aggravated by fatty-acid deficiency. When the balance of fatty acids is disturbed, so is cell membrane function. Whenever we assess detoxification patients with any kind of neurological toxicity syndrome, we check their fatty-acid levels to make sure that their bodies can repair the membrane damage.

This test is also useful for anyone who has a chronic or inflammatory illness.

The tests discussed in this chapter, and many others, can help you discover the true underlying causes of your health concerns. They represent a new way of thinking in the field—looking for problems that don't necessarily have names or that are precursors to known diseases. In functional medicine, it's not always necessary to label or name how you feel. What's important, however, is finding the correct tools for helping rebalance your biochemistry to make you feel better. Although you can still reap great benefits from detoxification without extensive lab work, these tests can really help.

CHAPTER 8

7-Day Detox Miracle

The EcoTox Program

- The First Step
- Health Safety: Who Should and Should Not Use This Program?
- How Often Should I Do This Program?
- The Three-Module Plan
- Module One: The Eco-Tox Detoxification Diet
- Making a Daily Plan
- Module Two: Supplementation
- Module Three: Circulation Therapy
- Summary: 7-Day Detox Program Guidelines
- Things to Do
- Obstacles to Your Week of Detoxification
- The Basic Detoxification Shopping List

Healing your body and achieving good health are much simpler than most of us imagine. We have a natural and miraculous capacity to self-heal and an inborn tendency toward health. In most situations, complex therapies aren't required. In a sense, all we need to do is get out of the way of our body's ability to detoxify and repair itself. A noted medical doctor named John H. Tilden wrote a book called *Toxemia Explained,* in which he detailed many recommendations that are used today by doctors in clinical detoxification programs. Joe Boucher, a well-known Canadian naturopathic physician, wrote, "The essence of all disease is the accumulation in the system of waste matter and impurities due to wrong habits of living. The elimination of this toxic matter from the body is what nature is striving for all the time. . . . It is through detoxification . . . that the healing latent within all of us can be given a free hand to function." Letting your body rest and taking a break from your regular schedule for one week allows all the organ systems dedicated to healing to undergo a change toward wellness.

Some simple methods are available that you can use to take care of yourself. The three health modules described in this chapter give you the basic tools that you need. After following this program for one week, you will feel better. Our clinical experience has conclusively proven that this week-long program is a winner. The basic program includes a detoxification diet, nutritional supplementation, hydrotherapy, and exercise. You'll begin to feel the benefits after about three days.

The first few days—what we call the initial "scrub" mode of internal cleansing—might be difficult for you, and during the seven days of the program you might feel hungry or weak. Unfortunately, this mild discomfort can't be avoided, but sit back, relax, and don't worry. These unpleasant sensations are a sign that the program is working and that your body is cleansing itself of toxic substances. Unless these difficulties are part of a separate disease process that has arisen at the same time, you should ignore the discomfort. Get as much rest as you feel you need and concentrate on completing all the exercises, following the instructions for hydrotherapy, and taking your supplements. If you have any questions or concerns about your symptoms, consult a health care practitioner.

Case History

Ray, a forty-year-old pastor, has always been interested in sports and nutrition. He came to us complaining of deteriorating teeth, mental fatigue, and exhaustion so severe he would almost faint while giving a sermon. A hair analysis revealed mineral deficiencies, and we recommended a specialized mineral supplement. We also asked him to do a seven-day detoxification program. Ray agreed and was surprised that energy improved immediately. He felt that he hadn't been able to be so active since he was in his twenties. By avoiding wheat, coffee, and sugar (which we identified as irritants for him), eating a proper diet, fasting regularly, and staying on his mineral supplement, Ray manages his own health, and no longer needs to see us.

All the following symptoms are considered a normal response to detoxification:

- Fatigue

- Headaches during the first three days

- Offensive body odor

- Sleep problems (insomnia or sleeping too much)

- Hunger

- Increased gas from extra vegetable fiber

- Bad breath

- Itchy skin

- Irritability

You can expect to see, to varying degrees, the following results from a detox program:

- Increased vitality, energy, and stamina

- Reduction of allergic symptoms

- Improvement of digestive functions

- Better concentration, clarity, and mental focus

- Enhanced mental performance

- A sense of calm and ease

- Increased resistance to illness

- Reduction in risk for many chronic diseases

- Reduced symptoms of chronic toxicity

- Weight loss

The First Step

The decision to take responsibility for healing yourself requires a burst of energy. It's a challenge to change your habits, especially in the beginning. The hardest part is to make the commitment to do something that requires planning, discipline, motivation, and a willingness to undergo some discomfort and inconvenience. If you could simply order the qualities needed for this effort from a catalog, you would need willpower and moral strength, a strong desire for vitality, a resolve to follow instructions, common sense, and a dedication to understanding your health program so that you're in full control of the process.

Healing can be hard work. Friends and family members can offer valuable support. In our practice, we see that when a family member agrees to go through the process with the patient, the rate and depth of the patient's healing accelerates and there's a better chance for a positive clinical outcome.

Ask a friend or family member to read this chapter with you. Make a plan for your detoxification week together. Ask him or her to help you organize all your supplements and food purchases. Make a date to eat together at least twice during your week so that you have some company and can socialize during mealtimes.

The EcoTox diet has been formulated for maximum digestibility. It's like eating without eating.

The success of this program, as well as your ability to self-heal, rests mainly on your resolve to focus on your health—now and in the future. As doctors, it has been our experience that this determination is closely linked to an individual's ability to acknowledge their own lack of well-being. Some of our patients become determined to change when they reach the point at which they're willing to do anything to escape the pain their disease is causing. The perception of pain, as unpleasant as it is, can become a powerful motivating force. If you're questioning your resolve to undertake this program, examine your life and ask yourself whether you're ignoring your discomfort—feelings that are really telling you that you have a problem that needs your attention. Unfortunately, no doctor can do this for you, and no medicine will make it any easier. To heal, each of us must face our weaknesses and commit to growing stronger—physically and emotionally.

Health Safety: Who Should and Should Not Use This Program?

The seven-day EcoTox program is safe for most people to use. As with any health regimen, specific reactions and results will vary from one individual to another, and effects that are considered normal vary widely. If you have any hesitation about your ability to undergo the rigor of detoxification, get a physical exam by your naturopathic or medical doctor. Request a blood chemistry screening to make sure that you're not anemic. Any history of liver or immune disorders might require special attention in the form of additional supplementation, as recommended by your doctor.

If you take any medications regularly, it's very important that you consult a health care professional before beginning the program. As you detoxify, the rate at which drugs are metabolized will change, and once the function of your body's mechanisms for detoxification have been revitalized, any drugs you're taking will be cleared from your bloodstream more quickly. This means that your dosage might need to be adjusted.

A word of warning: The seven-day EcoTox program is both safe and beneficial. However, some people shouldn't use this program by themselves. To minimize the risks of complications, we strongly recommend that people with certain specific diagnosed health conditions, as well as children and nursing mothers, work closely with a trained health care professional.

You need to seek professional assistance and use this program with a doctor's supervision if you:

- Have a terminal or malignant illness

- Have a genetic disease (an indication of an inherited metabolic problem)

- Have an autoimmune disease

- Are chronically underweight

- Suffer from hyperthyroidism

- Have a mental illness

- Take any medications regularly

- Are pregnant

How Often Should I Do This Program?

Probably the most frequent question posed to us on radio shows, in television interviews, and by newspaper reporters is, "How often should I do this program?" The answer to this question is simple: as often as you like. Some patients I see in the clinic who have autoimmune disease or cancer are placed on a program similar to ours on a permanent basis because of their weak immune systems. Because most of your immune system is in the liver and intestines, if you have any immune problems, by definition, you have an intestinal problem. Cancer patients benefit from a diet similar to the detox diet because they find simple foods easy to digest. Similarly, patients who consult me for a cold or flu are given a special diet like the detox diet. If the intestines are working overtime to deal with a diet that is irritating or difficult to digest, this will affect immune function throughout the whole body. An acute sinus infection is a good example. A sinus infection can be difficult to treat, even with antibiotics, because the patient is usually eating something that's irritating the intestines. When the patient changes his or her diet to rice, vegetables, and fruit for several weeks, the infection clears up. The sinuses are really just an extension of the digestive tract: By definition, chronic sinus problems are caused by chronic digestive problems.

You can do this program at least once a year, though several times a year is also probably a good idea. Anytime you feel run down, overstressed, sick, or whenever you experience headaches or the natural balance of your body goes out, you can do the program to reset your internal regulating mechanisms. When you rest the intestines, the healing machinery embedded in the liver and intestines goes into overdrive to help you recover optimum health.

The Three-Module Plan

The detox program consists of three modules. The first focuses on diet, the second on nutritional supplements, and the third on improving circulation through hydrotherapy and exercise. The recommendations offered for each module have been chosen to provide some variety so that you can pick and choose what best fits your situation. We urge you to use at least some recommendations from each module, but if the program in its entirety seems overwhelming, try focusing first on the diet module only. Follow the diet instructions precisely, as health begins in the aisles of your supermarket. Your overall health—present and future—depends on what happens in your digestive tract, what's in your refrigerator, and what's on your fork.

Module One: The EcoTox
Detoxification Diet

The foundation of the EcoTox plan is a specialized seven-day food plan. The first two days of the program prescribe a clear-liquid fast. No solid foods are consumed. Although this can be difficult and uncomfortable for some people, you will experience much better results if you start off this way. However, if you feel that fasting is more than you can cope with, you can modify the plan according to your needs by including some of the foods from the plan for the remaining five days.

For the first two days—preferably a weekend or days on which you don't need to go to work—consume only water, lemon water, herbal teas, and (if necessary) fresh juices (although the best results are obtained when juices aren't included). Going without food for two days poses no danger to your body. It's not uncommon for people to go without food for forty-eight hours when they're suffering from influenza, a fever, or a gastrointestinal infection. Your body has adequate food stores for two days of fasting.

Unlike many other detoxification regimens, we do not advocate a long-term juice or water fast. Our experience is that extended liquid fasts are too stressful for most people, although they can be excellent treatment programs for certain types of health problems when done under clinical supervision. A two-day liquid fast is a remarkably effective and safe method for cleaning the blood. Short liquid fasts have been successfully used for the treatment of pesticide poisoning, rheumatoid arthritis, pancreatitis, diabetes, heart disease, food allergy, irritable bowel syndrome, asthma, and psoriasis.

It's easy to become dehydrated without even knowing it. In our hyperactive society, many people ignore their thirst sensors and don't take the time to drink sufficient quantities of water each day. People often mistake thirst for hunger. We find dehydration especially prevalent in heavy coffee drinkers, who unknowingly are consuming a powerful diuretic that removes water from the body through the kidneys. Dehydration causes the accumulation of waste in the blood. The resulting blood toxicity has a profound effect on human health and metabolic efficiency. It is well known among runners that if you wait until you're thirsty to drink, you're already dehydrated and your performance decreases.

The compound D-limonene, found in the oil in the lemon peel, has been used to prevent and treat cancer in research animals. Its protective effects are due to its ability to induce Phases 1 and 2 detoxification to neutralize carcinogens. It also improves resistance to depletion of glutathione, a powerful detoxification agent.

During your week of detoxification, we recommend drinking a minimum of eight 8-ounce glasses of water daily. Choose distilled, filtered, or spring water—not tap water. Your water needs will vary with climate, temperature, and exercise: You need less water in a cold, damp climate and more water in a hot, dry climate, and generally you need more water with greater physical activity. Two quarts of water daily is a good baseline for everyone.

Lemon water is especially effective for rehydrating the body during this cleansing period. It can be drunk throughout the day instead of plain water (or in addition to it) during the liquid fast and for the following five days. You can drink lemon water hot or cold. To make it, simply take a quart of pure water and squeeze half an organically grown lemon into it. Add the remains of the lemon and the peel to the water and leave them there. If you need a little sweetener to make the lemon water more palatable, add half a cup of organic concord grape juice to a quart of lemon water.

During the two-day liquids-only fast, the filtering mechanisms of the liver can become overwhelmed. This can lead to sick feelings, much like those that accompany a fever. Taking the assigned supplements, including antioxidants (detailed in module two), helps prevent any side effects of enhanced liver detoxification, such as extreme fatigue, headaches, dizziness, hunger, offensive body odor, bad breath, and irritability. Some people find that they most benefit from taking no supplements at all during day fast—I find that a water-only fast is the easiest w

For people who can't afford to lose any weigh are in a debilitated condition, a protein shake two to three times a day during the first two days is recommended. In more severe cases of weakness, we suggest skipping the two days of fasting on liquids only and following the diet recommended here, which includes vegetables, fruit, and rice for seven days.

After the two-day fast, your diet for the remaining five days is simple: Eat fresh fruits, vegetables, and brown rice in any form. You can eat as much of these foods as you want, both cooked and uncooked.

Foods to Use

The following lists will help you plan your EcoTox diet. Remember that you can eat as much as you want of the permissible foods, except those for which quantities are specified. You must completely avoid all foods that are not permitted. You need to carefully read the labels on the packaged foods you buy to know exactly which ingredients they contain. Your best bet is to build your meals around fresh produce and brown rice. Organic produce, if available, is preferable. Shopping in a health food store will probably offer you more options than your local supermarket.

Carbohydrates *Use:* Brown rice, basmati rice, Thai (jasmine) rice, wild rice, and rice products such as rice cakes, rice crackers, breads and pasta made with rice flour (read the label to be sure they don't contain any wheat), and rice-based pancake mix. If you find that you need a break from rice, you can include the grains quinoa, amaranth, and millet as desired.

Avoid: Sugar, honey, molasses, artificial sweeteners, and all products containing them; corn and all products made with corn; and wheat and all products made with wheat or containing wheat gluten.

Legumes   *Use:* Mung beans, garbanzo beans (can be hard for some people to digest), bean thread noodles, and miso (a flavorful paste made of naturally fermented soybeans). *Avoid:* All other beans and products made with beans.

Vegetables and Fruits   *Use:* All varieties of fresh produce. The only exception is grapefruit, which shouldn't be eaten during this period because it contains a compound that inhibits liver detoxification. Fruits and vegetables can be steamed, baked, lightly sautéed in a small amount of virgin olive oil, eaten raw, or juiced. You can eat any vegetable combined with any other vegetable in any quantity you desire. Select from the following vegetables:

- Leafy green vegetables: lettuce (romaine, red, bib, mixed leaf), spinach, endive, kale, chard, bok choy, escarole, arugula

- Root vegetables: carrots, beets, potatoes, sweet potatoes, yams, celery root, parsnips, parsley root, radishes (including their green leafy tops), turnips, rutabagas

- Cruciferous vegetables: cabbage, cauliflower, broccoli, brussels sprouts, mustard greens

- Vine vegetables: cucumbers, zucchini, and all other varieties of squash

- Onion family: shallots, garlic, onions, leeks

- Others: asparagus; celery; okra; artichoke (Jerusalem and globe); eggplant; string beans; red, green, yellow and orange peppers; seaweed; kelp; naturally fermented sauerkraut with no added vinegar or preservatives

Raw vegetable salads are difficult for some people to digest. You should steam and bake your vegetables if you experience digestive discomfort. Raw foods are an excellent source of vitamins, enzymes, and minerals, but if you can't digest them, you shouldn't eat them. Fresh pressed fruit and vegetable juices are also a wonderful alternative. They offer all the life energy of raw foods but are easier on the digestive system.

Initially, you might notice an increase in intestinal gas from the increased consumption of vegetables. This is the result of bacterial fermentation of plant cell wall products, but it should gradually dissipate. If problems with gas persist, stick to lightly steamed vegetables and stay away from raw vegetable salads, cabbage, and onions. You can also reduce gas by using ginger root and powder, cardamom, and cinnamon to season your food. Indian and Ayurvedic cookbooks feature recipes with carminative spices to help with digestive discomfort and decrease gas.

The following fruits and vegetables typically cause problems for some people, including hives, wheezing, headaches, and stomach upset. Avoid *only* those that bother you:

- Apples
- Carrots
- Onions
- Green and red peppers
- Raspberries
- Plums
- Mangoes
- Oranges
- Melons (all varieties)
- Tomatoes
- Garlic
- Eggplant
- Cucumbers
- Cherries
- Papayas
- Fresh figs
- Strawberries

Fats and Oils   *Use:* Olive oil (extra virgin) or unheated flaxseed oil (only 2 tablespoons daily).

Avoid: All other oils and forms of fat, including butter and margarine.

If organic produce is not available, wash foods well.
To remove pesticides, you can use one of the following
methods:

1. Fill a sink with cold water plus a few drops of PURE
   castille soap (available at most health food stores).
   Dip fruits and vegetables in the solution, scrub with
   a vegetable brush, and rinse.

2. Soak fruits and vegetables in a sink half-filled with
   cold water plus 1 tablespoon of 35 percent food-grade
   hydrogen peroxide for five to fifteen minutes. The
   shorter time is for thin-skinned and soft fruits and leafy
   vegetables; the longer time is for heavy-skinned, fi-
   brous, and root vegetables and hard and thick-skinned
   fruits. Rinse thoroughly in fresh water after soaking.

3. Soak fruits and vegetables in 1 gallon of cold water
   plus 1 teaspoon of unscented Clorox Regular bleach.
   This type of bleach is the only one that doesn't contain harmful additives: Don't use any other form or
   brand. Follow the soaking times for method two.
   Then rinse for five minutes under fresh, cold running water. Avoid grapes and strawberries if they
   aren't organic.

Beverages   *Use:* Herbal teas, green tea, water, lemon water, diluted fruit juices, vegetable juices, water (only filtered, spring,
or distilled).

   Avoid: Coffee, black teas, and all forms of alcohol, including beer and wine.

Condiments   *Use:* Vegetable salt, sea salt, vinegar, naturally
fermented soy sauce or tamari, any culinary spices, and
miso.

Avoid: Ketchup, mayonnaise, Worcestershire sauce, barbecue sauce, and all other packaged relishes, dressings, and seasonings.

Foods to Avoid

The foods that form the basis of a normal Western diet cause the liver to work overtime as it tries to metabolize the dense concentration of nutrients that are constantly flooding the digestive system and bloodstream. Poor digestion is one of the main causes of toxicity because it adds an unnecessary and in many cases overwhelming burden to the liver's normal workload. The liver simply can't keep up with the quantity of contaminants in the blood that must be processed. When food is properly digested, the liver can attend to its job of detoxification. The EcoTox diet has been formulated for maximum digestibility. It's like eating without eating. This is why it's essential to avoid all the following foods:

- Meat, fish, poultry, and eggs

- Dairy products

- Fats and oils (other than the recommended amount of 2 tablespoons daily of extra virgin olive oil or flaxseed oil)

- Chocolate

- Nuts

- Beans (other than mung beans and any listed soybean-based products)

- Grains (other than rice, quinoa, amaranth, and millet)

- Foods made with flour from wheat, corn, and oats

- Sugar

- Alcohol

- Coffee and black teas

A Word on Rice

Because it's a light food that digests easily while supplying carbohydrate energy essential for daily activity, brown rice is perfect for detoxification. You can boil it, bake it, fry it (with only 1 tablespoon of olive oil daily), and put it in soup. Rice is unequaled as a food for curing many of the diseases induced by Western diets.

Most people digest rice easily. For some, the lighter rices, such as basmati or Thai, are easier on their digestive systems than brown rice. In the literature of medical research, rice is an accepted hypoallergenic food. This means that it rarely stimulates or aggravates allergic reactions. Rice is gluten-free, and in one study of seven hundred atopic patients (people genetically predisposed to certain allergies) only 1 percent showed sensitivity. Historically, rice diets have been used in Western medicine to manage diarrhea in adults and children. Studies show that rice has been used in the treatment of children with diarrhea to enhance superior healing. In addition, it's high in an antioxidant called ferulic acid. Ferulic acid has been studied in the treatment of a variety of inflammatory bowel disorders and has been found to have a remarkable ability to prevent inflammation in the intestinal membranes.

When people are discouraged about how restrictive the EcoTox diet is, we try to cheer them up by reminding them that most Asian cultures live on rice, eating it three times a day. Having to subsist on rice, fruits, and vegetables for one week might seem like a plan for starvation, but this is the normal daily diet for millions of people around the world. Not only will it do you no harm, it will allow your detoxification mechanisms to work more effectively and give the blood-cleaning filters of the body an opportunity to catch up and clear out the overload of toxins that have accumulated.

Your food choices are limited, but relax: After the two-day water fast, it's only for five days.

Food Is Good Medicine

Eating a large quantity of vegetables and rice every day, after the initial two-day liquid fast, is a big change for those who are used to eating a great deal of bread, pasta, and meat. However, by being creative in your food preparation, you might find the change more enjoyable than you expect. In addition, a visit to your local farmers' market or a walk through the produce department of a good supermarket will reveal a huge variety to choose from. The following are some foods that you should be sure to include in your detox diet—and regularly in your meals after your detox week—because they offer special healing benefits.

Beets Daily portions of beets, an excellent source of betaine, are good for the blood, intestines, and liver. In our clinic, we notice that beets keep our patients regular, especially while they're going through the detoxification program. Eating beets every day is a safe way to alleviate constipation, both acute and chronic. In addition, beets have long been used as a folk remedy for liver disorders, as betaine is essential for proper liver function and fat metabolism. Research has found that betaine protects the liver from the ravages of excessive alcohol consumption, making it an important substance for detoxification. It has no known harmful effects and should be considered a dietary substance that has medicinal benefits, a safe and effective food "drug" for a toxic liver and for other toxic conditions.

Betaine has proven helpful in the management of homocysteinemia, a disorder involving altered amino acid metabolism. Although usually an inherited genetic condition, homocysteinemia can also be brought on by a diet high in red meat combined with deficiencies in folic acid and vitamins B_{12} and B_6. The body has difficulty breaking down a molecule called homocysteine, which, as it builds up in the blood, initiates the destruction of blood vessels and damages the artery walls, increasing one's susceptibility to cardiovascular disease. (Many medical experts now believe that elevated blood levels of homocysteine, not high cholesterol, are the main cause of cardiovascular disease in Western society.)

The success of this program, as well as your ability to self-heal, rests mainly on your resolve to focus on your health—now and in the future.

Homocysteinemia responds to vitamin supplementation, but betaine supplementation is often overlooked even though it's especially important for patients who are genetically prone to produce an excess of homocysteine. The betaine found in beets is an important source of a molecule that accelerates the detoxification of homocysteine and transforms it into cysteine, a safe amino acid.

Broccoli Cruciferous vegetables, a group that includes broccoli, brussels sprouts, cabbage, and cauliflower, offer the body special protection. All are high in a unique class of substances called glucosinolates. These are used to make compounds, such as indole-3-carbinol, sulforaphane, and cyanohydroxybutene, which researchers believe improve the ability of the liver and other organs to detoxify drugs, chemicals, and pollutants.

Broccoli sprouts have the highest concentration of these protective substances. They have been shown to change the rate of liver detoxification so that toxins in the blood can be cleared more easily. The therapeutic potential of these natural antioxidants is so powerful that the pharmaceutical industry is looking at ways to synthesize them to create a new class of food drugs called phytochemicals. Science has finally caught up with mothers, who have long urged their children to eat their vegetables.

Green Barley Powder   One food that has been shown to counteract the negative effect of intestinal poisons is green barley powder. Barley shoot extract is nature's ideal antioxidant. The flavonoids that it contains protect against cell membrane damage caused by toxins. This can be especially helpful in the intestines. The bioflavonoid 2-0-GIV has antioxidant capabilities that outperform vitamin E and BHT. In the clinic, we have had several patients with advanced bowel disease experience excellent results with green barley extract.

Artichokes and Other Inulin Foods   Inulin, a substance found in artichokes, Jerusalem artichokes, and burdock root, is a powerful stimulator of the kidneys and the immune system, and daily portions of these vegetable are very helpful during the detoxification process. Elecampane, echinacea, and sunflower also contain high amounts of inulin.

Historically, all these foods and herbs have been used as blood cleansers, and we now understand that a real scientific basis exists for the tradition. Poisons from harmful bowel bacteria (endotoxins) tend to leak into the bloodstream and wreak havoc on the detoxification mechanisms of the liver. Inulin-containing foods and plants turn on a part of the immune system called the alternate complement pathway. When this chemical switch is turned on, the body intensifies its efforts to clear out these bacterial poisons.

Rice Protein Research has shown that protein plays an important role in tissue detoxification. To add high-quality protein to your five-day plan and alleviate hunger and the difficulty of eating away from home, we recommend a shake made with rice protein concentrate. The powder is mixed with juice or water, and fresh fruit can also be blended into the shake. You can drink a rice protein shake several times a day, in mid-morning and mid-afternoon as a snack, and as a meal replacement. Some people have a high biological need for protein. If you experience extreme fatigue that's not alleviated by sleep once you begin the diet, it's especially important for you to include rice protein concentrate.

Liquid protein drinks have been used for years by medical doctors in the treatment of food allergy and food intolerance. These drinks contain no intact dietary protein but utilize free-form amino acids and fatty acids, vitamins, and minerals. Unlike other protein shake formulas that often taste unpleasant, rice protein concentrates are more palatable. In addition, medical research has shown that most people can tolerate rice protein concentrates, which are hypoallergenic. Some detoxification programs suggest consuming only rice protein shakes for several weeks. In the EcoTox program, the rice protein shake is used as a snack during the first two days or as an occasional meal replacement. In our clinic, we put patients on an exclusive diet of rice protein concentrate formula only if they're quite ill.

Ultra Clear, developed by Healthcomm Inc., is an extremely popular, patented, rice protein product and is ideal for detoxification therapy. In one study using this product, it was found that patients were 53 percent improved in liver detoxification tests. In another study, patients using Ultra Clear had a 52 percent reduction in toxicity symptoms on their symptom questionnaire scores, as well as an improvement on liver detoxification function and intestinal permeability. Ultra Clear contains supplemental NAC, glutathione, glutamine, inulin, and the full spectrum of vitamin nutrients we recommend. The product also contains medium chain triglycerides. This type of fat, which is quickly absorbed and efficiently used by the body, increases energy production for the purpose of detoxification. Ultra Clear is available only through health care professionals. (For information about how your health care provider can order Ultra Clear, see the Healthcomm Web site at www.healthcomm.com.) A number of other brands of rice protein concentrate are available in most health food stores, including a product distributed by Nutribiotic. For more product information, visit our Web site at www.peterbennett.com.

Common Problems on the Detox Program and Their Antidotes

The ten most common problems you'll experience during your seven days and antidotes to these problems are the following:

1. Dizziness. Cause: low blood sugar. Antidote: increase fluids and rice intake.

2. Nausea. Cause: bile stagnation. Antidote: strong lemon and water with a pinch of cayenne pepper on waking.

3. Constipation. Cause: lowered food intake. Antidote: increase flaxseed powder in the rice protein shakes.

4. Excessive weight loss. Cause: lowered calorie intake in individuals with high metabolic rates. Antidote: increase oil (olive/flax) intake.

5. Diarrhea. Cause: increased fiber intake from fruits and vegetables. Antidote: this usually lasts only several days and can be offset by eating more rice.

6. Headaches. Cause: dehydration, caffeine withdrawal, liver congestion. Antidote: increase water intake and hot and cold showering on the back of the head.

7. Insomnia. Cause: low blood sugar and liver congestion. Antidote: fruit shake before bed.

8. Hunger. Cause: low calorie intake. Antidote: rice protein shakes two or three times a day.

9. Intestinal gas. Cause: increased vegetable fiber intake. Antidote: one charcoal tablet after each meal.

10. Irritability/fatigue/dullness. Cause: low calorie intake. Antidote: rice protein shakes two or three times a day.

Making a Daily Plan

Days One and Two

Consume water, lemon water, and herbal tea only, as often as you want. Be sure to meet your minimum daily requirement of eight 8-ounce glasses of liquids.

Days Three Through Seven

The following is what a typical day's menu might look like (variations depend on your appetite and preferences). You might need to eat more or less than this amount of food. Include snacks only if you find yourself hungry between meals. Remember that thirst is often mistaken for hunger.

Upon arising: 8 ounces of hot lemon water

Breakfast: A rice protein shake made with fresh fruit and fruit juice; rice cakes; fresh fruit; herbal tea

Snack: Fruit and/or a protein shake; herbal tea

Lunch: Salad and soup; rice and steamed vegetables; baked or sweet potato and cold steamed vegetables

Snack: Fruit and/or protein shake; rice cakes; rice crackers; herbal tea

Dinner: Rice and mixed vegetables, steamed or lightly sautéed; soup and salad; salad and baked potato

Day Eight

On the morning of the eighth day, begin adding protein into your diet. After the seven days of restricted foods, you use this period to gradually add foods into your diet and try to determine if some foods you were eating were upsetting the digestive system and liver. You can be "sensitive" to foods and not allergic; the result is an ongoing irritation in your digestive tract and immune system that weakens your overall vitality.

I recommend, as your first new food, that you begin with eggs because they are a perfect protein from the standpoint of amino acid balance. However, some people are allergic to eggs or do not tolerate them and so should not use them as the first food. Those who do not tolerate the eggs (symptoms are gallbladder pain, stomach pain, abdominal burning, or sulfur burps) will move on to the next step, which is to begin adding fish or fowl (chicken or turkey). This should be done over three to four days. Vegetarians who do not eat animal sources of protein should move on to the next step by adding other foods. Many of the patients seen in our clinic who have been long-term vegetarians and are not healthy (weight gain, fatigue, muscle soreness, or poor concentration) are advised at this step to try adding animal protein at this time to see if they feel better.

Food Testing

Test one new food each day. It may take weeks to get through all the food testing listed here, and it is not necessarily important for all individuals. Those with the following problems should go through the complete food testing program:

Psychological: Anxiety, depression, insomnia, food cravings, childhood attention deficit disorder

Ear, Nose, and Throat: Chronic nasal congestion, teeth grinding, postnasal drip, chronic fluid in the ears, Meniere's syndrome (chronic dizziness)

Gastrointestinal: Irritable bowel syndrome, constipation, diarrhea, abdominal cramping, ulcerative colitis, Crohn's disease, gallbladder disease, infantile colic

Cardiovascular: High blood pressure, arrhythmia, angina, edema

Skin: Acne, eczema, psoriasis, canker sores (aphthous ulcers), hives

Musculoskeletal: Muscle aches, osteoarthritis, rheumatoid arthritis

Neurologic: Migraines and other headaches, numbness

Respiratory: Asthma, recurrent colds, sore throats, ear infections

Urogenital: Urinary tract infections, prostate inflammation, yeast infections, bed wetting, frequent urination

Metabolic: Obesity

If one of your problems is arthritis, test one new food every other day because joint pain reactions may be delayed. Also remember to test pure sources of a food. For example, do not use pizza to test cheese because pizza also contains wheat and corn oil.

Dairy tests: Test milk and then cheese on a separate day. You may wish to try several cheeses on different days because some people are sensitive to one cheese but not another. Test yogurt, cottage cheese, or butter separately.

Wheat test: Use a pure wheat cereal.

Corn test: Use fresh ears of corn or frozen corn (without sauces or preservatives).

Citrus test: Oranges, grapefruits, lemons, and limes. Test these individually on four separate days. The lemon and lime can be squeezed into Perrier or seltzer. With oranges and grapefruit, use the whole fruit.

Food additive test: Buy a set of food dyes and colors. Put half a teaspoon of each color in a glass. Add 1 teaspoon of the mixture to a glass of pineapple juice or diluted (50:50 with water) grape juice. This is especially helpful for children with hyperactivity and behavior disorders.

After you've discovered which foods you are sensitive to, challenge them several times to confirm that the food is disturbing to your body. Then make a commitment to not eat that food for six months before retesting it again.

Diet Tips and Guidelines

The following are some general tips to help you with the diet and to help you avoid toxins found in places you might not expect. We strongly recommend continuing these practices even after your detoxification week.

- Some individuals feel weak on this detox diet. This is because of the low amino acid (protein) and carbohydrate intake. If this is interfering with your work, first try adding more rice or root vegetables. If this doesn't help, take an extra rice protein shake during the day.

- Prepare your own homemade soup and make enough for a few meals. Use vegetable stock or water rather than chicken or beef stock. Instant miso soup is available at most health food stores.

- Be sure to use only stainless steel, glass, cast iron, or enameled steel cooking utensils and food storage containers. Avoid aluminum and plastic.

- It will be to your advantage to use natural products: natural herbal deodorants that don't contain aluminum, nonfluoridated toothpaste made with baking soda, and all natural soaps and shampoos.

- Avoid exposure to cleaning solutions, solvents, and chemicals.

This diet program has proven to be the easiest to follow and the least expensive of any other we have tried. In our practice, it has had the lowest relapse and dropout rate. The design of the program is the result of many years of personal and clinical research. We have studied much of the medical literature on the subject, observed many patients as they followed a variety of detoxification recommendations, and, most important, have tried many different detoxification dietary regimens ourselves. We're convinced that the plan we've created offers the best of all solutions to a wide variety of health problems.

Module Two: Supplementation

Your nutritional needs during the detoxification process are quite high. Shortages of critical nutrients can inhibit or even arrest entire biochemical pathways, thus making some patients dangerously toxic when they go without food for more than a few days. Without proper nutritional supplementation, it's possible to feel quite ill. A person who is already sick with a toxicity syndrome has even greater nutritional requirements. The body uses a number of methods to remove toxins, and, operating with an ecological perspective, we believe that it's essential to support the whole body and all its functions simultaneously.

For thousands of years, herbs, clays, and special substances have been used to assist in purifying the body and supporting it during detoxification, especially those that stimulated and protected the liver. Scientific research has identified new remedies to be used in detoxification, such as the mineral molybdenum and the amino acid n-acetyl-cysteine. Today, our knowledge of biochemistry makes it possible to understand why traditional remedies are effective and to choose from hundreds of detoxification medicines. Taking the best of both the old and the new, we list a range of therapeutic options that include traditional elements and the latest biochemical approaches.

As you detoxify, the rate at which drugs are metabolized will change.

In general, nutritional supplementation should fulfill the following key functions in a detoxification program:

- Protect body tissues from the volatile chemical products generated during the molecular "demolition" that accompanies internal cleansing

- Assist in the breakdown of toxins so that they are more readily eliminated

- Increase the flow of bile from the liver

- Facilitate the excretion of bile from the intestinal tract

- Reseed the intestines with favorable bacteria

- Heal damaged bowel membranes

- Purge the bowels

- Nourish all systems and organs

Each of these functions represents what we call a detoxification strategy group, and we recommend that everyone use at least one substance from each group.

Strategy Group One: Antioxidants for Tissue Protection

Antioxidant nutrients protect the tissues. The most well-known antioxidants are vitamins C and E. Less familiar but equally important antioxidants include lipoic acid and milk thistle. The general opinion of nutritionally oriented physicians is to provide a full range of all the antioxidants whenever using them in therapy. Let's discuss these antioxidants in some detail.

Vitamin C   Vitamin C is an essential nutrient that affects most body functions. Orthomolecular physicians, medical doctors who specialize in the use of vitamins and minerals for the treatment of disease, have been using high doses of vitamin C for many years to reverse acute and chronic disease. Vitamin C plays critical roles in numerous body systems. It activates white blood cells called neutrophils and the production of lymphocytes in the immune system. It is involved in fat metabolism and the absorption of iron. It works with enzymes and helps with the conversion of the amino acid tryptophan to the neurotransmitter serotonin (the so-called "feel-good" brain chemical). Collagen, the basic substance of connective tissue, is an essential component of tissue regeneration. Vitamin C is important in collagen tissue formation.

Many conditions in the body, including inflammation and detoxification, increase the production of free radicals. That is why protective substances for free radicals are called antioxidants; that is, they act to protect cells from harmful oxygen variants. As an antioxidant, vitamin C helps check the production of free radicals, protecting vulnerable cellular structures from the damage they cause.

Toxic metals, such as lead, mercury, and aluminum, can be chelated out of the body using vitamin C. In chelation, heavy metals bind with the vitamin molecules and are carried out of the body. Megadoses of vitamin C are very effective in cases of mercury poisoning and should be considered an essential component of mercury detoxification therapy. Some dentists recommend intravenous vitamin C during silver amalgam removal to prevent the mercury released in the drilling process from interfering with cellular enzymes and being absorbed into body tissues.

Vitamin C is an excellent bacteriostatic (meaning it prevents the growth of viruses and bacteria) and should be considered by all doctors and patients as a first line of therapeutic defense in cases of infection. To be effective, high enough doses must be used. Studies have shown that vitamin C can neutralize a wide variety of bacterial toxins, including tetanus, diphtheria, and staph. It also has proven helpful in defending against tuberculosis, a common infection sixty years ago that has lately reemerged in forms with a tendency to resist current, and toxic, drug therapy.

Vitamin C appears to be a kind of universal antitoxin, although researchers haven't yet identified the precise mechanism by which it exerts its influence over a wide variety of toxic substances. Studies have shown it to be effective against snake venom, chemicals such as benzene, and strychnine (a plant toxin). This suggests that vitamin C can protect us from toxins in plants and animals, as well as industrial chemicals. No other known compound possesses such a range of protective properties. Its universal application, safety, and low cost make it unequaled in the pharmaceutical industry.

Despite some reports to the contrary, the safety of vitamin C in large doses has been confirmed both in the laboratory and in the clinical setting. The fear that at high doses vitamin C caused kidney stones has proven unfounded. The experience of many clinicians with thousands of patients demonstrates that there is no danger of forming kidney stones when large doses of vitamin C are administered. Certain occupational exposures and lifestyle habits increase the daily need for vitamin C. For example, smoking depletes the body's stores of vitamin C, diminishing the body's ability to get rid of the harmful chemicals that it is exposed to in daily life. In our clinic, vitamin C is regarded as the most important supplement for detoxification.

The starting dose we usually recommend for the Eco-Tox detoxification program is 2 g of vitamin C, three times daily. If this doesn't loosen the bowels within one or two days, increase the dosage 1 g every day until well tolerated by the bowel. For serious problems like acute infections and toxic poisoning, start with 1 g every hour. If this does not cause diarrhea, double this dose. Individuals vary in how much vitamin C their bodies can comfortably handle. In some cases patients can take up to 20 g of vitamin C daily without any negative effect on the bowels. Clinical observation confirms that tolerance for such high doses is indicative of a patient's physiological need. We have some patients who can handle only 250 mg daily. Sometimes the type of vitamin C is important. The most easily tolerated type for preventing diarrhea is sodium ascorbate.

We recommend that you work up to 4 to 20 g of vitamin C daily. This dosage can be continued following your detoxification week. It can be especially helpful if your occupation exposes you to pollutants or industrial chemicals.

Vitamin E   Vitamin E is a fat-soluble vitamin discovered in 1922 by Herbert Evan and Katherine Bishop. It's an important antioxidant for detoxification as it offers protection from cell membrane lipid peroxidation. The process of detoxification can create dangerous molecules. Unless these "renegade molecules" are controlled, they can do more damage than the original toxin. Cell membrane damage by free radicals generated during detoxification has been associated with cardiovascular disease, cancer, nervous system disorders, immune system dysfunction, cataracts, and arthritis. Vitamin E also helps to stabilize blood glucose and prevents muscle tissue breakdown.

The recommended dosage of vitamin E is 200 to 1,200 IU daily. *Note:* Taking more than the recommended dosage of vitamin E is not necessarily better. A recent study looked at the effects of varying amounts of vitamin E. After twenty weeks, it was shown that doses of vitamin E can be helpful, but larger doses did not seem to offer significantly more protection unless there was tremendous oxidative stress, as in smokers or those exposed to chemical pollutants.

Glutathione Reduced glutathione (GSH) is a major antioxidant and free-radical scavenger. Glutathione is an essential component of liver detoxification. It's remarkable because it can do two jobs in the detoxification cycle: It intercepts toxic compounds from Phase 1 detoxification, and it combines with Phase 2 toxic chemicals to form a water-soluble conjugate that can be excreted in the bile and urine. Because glutathione is not broken down easily by digestive enzymes in the intestines, it's available to intestinal cells for local "first pass" detoxification. Therefore, oral supplementation is not the best way to increase glutathione in the body.

The body must manufacture glutathione from other amino acids in the liver for more efficient detoxification in the blood. It is found in fruits and vegetables and is assembled in the body from the amino acids glycine, cysteine, and glutamic acid. Glutathione deficiency comes from poor diet, free-radical stress, and toxic overload.

Although studies have demonstrated the effectiveness of glutathione supplementation in some conditions, we feel that boosting glutathione levels, other than by dietary means, is not a good idea. Eating fresh fruits and vegetables provides adequate glutathione for localized intestinal detoxification. For blood cleansing, we suggest using other precursor substances that seem to be better absorbed than glutathione. Research has shown that when comparisons are made between cost and tissue saturation, doses of oral vitamin C are cheaper and more effective than supplemental glutathione. N-acetyl-cysteine is also effective in boosting blood levels of glutathione.

For many patients who have problems with severe toxicity, central nervous system damage, kidney disease, and cardiovascular disease, I have been using intravenous glutathione with excellent results. Because it does not absorb well from the gut, the intravenous route has shown promise as a powerful way to offer protection to the body with a tool that is fast and effective. Two interesting medical studies have been published showing dramatic results with intravenous glutathione. One study showed that patients benefited from intravenous glutathione after a heart attack. Another study was done in Italy by a neurologist who showed that intravenous glutathione (600 mg twice daily) significantly improved patients with early Parkinson's disease (42 percent decline in disability).

The recommended dosage of glutathione consists of daily servings of fresh fruits and vegetables.

Lipoic Acid   Lipoic acid is an element found in foods rich in B-complex vitamins, such as liver and yeast. When you are shopping for lipoic acid, it has so many different names, like alpha-lipoic acid, thioctic acid, biletan, lipoicin, thioctacid, and thioctan, that you may have trouble finding it. Your body makes small amounts of lipoic acid, so it is not a true vitamin and is not essential in our diet. Unfortunately, there is not much information on the food sources of this nutrient. But foods that contain mitochondria, especially red meats, are thought to provide the highest levels of alpha-lipoic acid.

Lipoic acid is unusual because it's both an antioxidant and a B-vitamin-like substance. It is also a potent antioxidant in both fat- and water-soluble mediums, which is an unusual property. Its antioxidant abilities extend to both the oxidized and the reduced form. This is like having a football player who can play offense and defense equally well. Lipoic acid turns out to be a vitamin-like "universal antioxidant." It helps other antioxidants, like vitamin C, vitamin E, co-enzyme Q_{10}, and glutathione, to "recharge" themselves to their active forms.

Cells in your body use lipoic acid to generate energy. Therefore, it helps improve energy metabolism, especially in individuals who are chronically ill. Like other liver-protecting agents, lipoic acid has proven effective in treating poisoning from mercury, lead, carbon tetrachloride, and aniline dyes. It has also been used to treat liver disease and alcohol-induced cirrhosis. It's a potent antioxidant and should be considered when treating viral hepatitis, AIDS, glaucoma, and complications of diabetes.

The use of lipoic acid for diabetics is compelling. Research shows that it reverses the glycation (hardening) of protein caused by elevated blood glucose, which is believed to contribute to many of the complications seen in diabetes. These glycated proteins are referred to as advanced glycosylation end products (AGEs) and are thought to be responsible for the kidney damage and advanced atherosclerosis seen in diabetes.

Clinically, I have seen remarkable results in patients undergoing detoxification medicine who use lipoic acid. They recover more quickly. I believe that lipoic acid is an extremely important supplement for this program.

The recommended dosage of lipoic acid is 600 mg twice daily.

Strategy Group Two: Amino Acids for the Breakdown of Toxins

An amino acid is an organic compound that, when bonded together in chemical chains, forms the proteins that are the fundamental components of all living cells and plays a vital role in the growth and repair of tissues. Enzymes, hormones, and antibodies that are essential for the proper functioning of the body are made from protein; the amino acids from which these proteins are built can be obtained from foods such as meat, fish, eggs, milk, and legumes.

Amino acids have a special ability to "grasp" toxins in the body, capturing them and facilitating their removal. Studies show that patients who have a protein deficiency can't access the critical amino acids needed for detoxification. Their livers become sluggish, resulting in a toxic buildup in their bodies. People with a consistently low intake of dietary protein, including vegetarians and vegans, increase their risk of toxicity from exposure to environmental pollution and other toxic syndromes.

Because laboratory results have shown the damaging effects of low-protein diets and amino acid deficiencies for patients undergoing detoxification, we recommend glycine, n-acetyl-cysteine, and methionine supplementation to all patients to prevent any possibility of a shortage of these critical amino acids and to facilitate detoxification. We strongly advocate including all these amino acids in your detox program, but of the three, the most important supplement to include is n-acetyl-cysteine (NAC). Let's take a closer look at NAC and some other important amino acids.

NAC NAC is the primary precursor to glutathione, a liver compound that drives the mechanism for shuttling toxins out of the body. Studies have shown that NAC affects concentrations of glutathione in the blood, helping to provide adequate levels so that the chemicals produced during detoxification don't damage other tissues.

NAC is easily absorbed in the digestive tract and is six times more cost effective than supplemental glutathione. Clinical studies have shown that NAC has demonstrated the following properties:

- It's safe.

- It's an effective free-radical quencher and fairly resistant to oxidation.

- It boosts glutathione production.

- It prevents mucus in the lungs.

- It's useful in the treatment of overdose syndromes from substances such as acetaminophen.

- It increases immune responses.

- It's useful for AIDS patients because of its ability to replenish glutathione.

- It helps regulate liver-detoxifying amino acids, such as sulfate, taurine, and glutathione.

The recommended dosage of NAC is 500 mg three times daily between meals.

Note: Any intestinal yeast infections should be eliminated prior to NAC therapy.

Glycine Glycine is a nonessential amino acid that the body uses for detoxification reactions in the liver (explained in chapter 5). In the 1930s, a medical doctor named Armand Quick had good results using glycine for his patients with liver disease. Roger Williams, the renowned and visionary biochemist, was one of the early advocates of nutritional medicine for the treatment of disease and promoted glycine supplementation for alcoholics in the 1950s.

Not only is glycine a necessary component of the detoxification pathway in the liver, but it's also a building block for glutathione, the most vigorous free-radical scavenger in the body. Glycine is considered a conditionally essential nutrient. This means that only under certain conditions is the body's need for glycine likely to exceed production or dietary availability. When these conditions arise, as during periods of detoxification, the supplementation of glycine has shown to be beneficial.

The recommended dosage of glycine is 1,500 to 3,000 mg daily between meals.

Methionine   We were taught in naturopathic medical school that methionine is essential as a lipotropic. These are substances that increase the removal of fat in the liver. Lipotropics, including methionine, are usually molecule donors, which means they contribute a particular type of molecule that is needed in certain detoxification reactions. Other lipotropic agents are choline, betaine (remember the beets?), folic acid, and vitamin B_{12}. Herbs that have the properties of cholagogues, meaning that they stimulate the contraction of the gallbladder, and choleretics, meaning that they stimulate bile secretion in the liver, are usually also thought of as lipotropics (for more details on choleretics and cholagogues, see "Strategy Group Three: Bile Lubricants").

In addition to its role in fat metabolism, methionine performs many other critical jobs in the body. It combines with the cellular fuel ATP to form S-adenosylmethionine (SAM), the main source of methyl groups. Methyl groups are very important for cellular biochemical reactions. Methionine is used in RNA and DNA and in the production of taurine and cysteine, two other critical detoxification amino acids. Methionine is especially important in breaking down estrogen, making it very important in the treatment of premenstrual syndrome (PMS), which can be caused by a toxic excess of estrogen hormones.

The metabolism of methionine depends on the presence of adequate levels of vitamins B_6 and B_{12} and folic acid. Without vitamins B_6 and B_{12}, there's a buildup of homocysteine in the blood. This buildup is known as a folate trap. Anyone who is taking methionine or eating a diet high in methionine (for example, a meat diet) needs to supplement with extra folic acid and vitamins B_6 and B_{12}.

Some experts feel that those who have poor sulfoxidation abilities, usually due to a genetic metabolic defect, should avoid methionine supplementation, believing that it can cause a toxic buildup in the bloodstream of the amino acid cysteine, which could eventually affect the nervous system. This defect is related to another defect resulting in low availability in the enzyme sulfite oxidase. To determine whether you have this defect, ask your doctor to test your sulfite oxidase levels. Symptoms of sulfite oxidase insufficiencies are headaches, chronic pain, gastrointestinal problems, and a history of reactions to sulfite-containing foods. If you find you have high urinary sulfites, you can treat your problem with supplementation of extra molybdenum.

The recommended dosage of methionine is 1,000 mg two or three times daily.

Strategy Group Three: Bile Lubricants

A tried-and-true method for internal cleansing among naturopathic physicians is to use natural remedies to increase bile flow. Toxins are excreted from the liver through bile fluid, and when the flow is stimulated and improved, the liver can remove poisons more effectively. Dandelion root (taraxacum), turmeric, chelidonium, artichokes, lecithin, ox bile salts, and milk thistle are excellent bile lubricants. You don't need all these bile lubricants, however, so select just one from the following list:

Taraxacum Dandelion root is high in the compound inulin (discussed earlier in this chapter). The benefits of dandelion come from its ability to increase bile production and simultaneously activate the gallbladder to excrete it. Dandelion is a safe, gentle, and effective bile lubricant and should be used in relatively high doses.

The recommended dosage of dandelion root is 1 teaspoon of solid extract three times daily or 8 g daily of powdered root as a tea.

Turmeric Turmeric is a common spice in South Asian cuisine. Its distinctive yellow color is a defining characteristic of Indian curries. Although not a spice with general appeal to a Western palate, turmeric is very important as a medicine. It has been used by Indian and Chinese healers for thousands of years to protect the liver and promote bile flow. The therapeutic agent in turmeric is thought to be curcumin, a bioflavonoid contained in turmeric's yellow pigment.

Current research has identified turmeric as a powerful anti-inflammatory, comparable in effectiveness to any anti-inflammatory drug currently on the market. Studies have shown it to be especially helpful in the management of arthritis pain. Curcumin's ability to fight inflammation also makes it helpful as an antioxidant, scavenging free radicals and protecting DNA from oxidant breakage and lipid peroxidation.

The recommended dosage of turmeric is 4 capsules after every meal or 1 teaspoon stirred into a cup of warm liquid after every meal. (You can make your own curcumin capsules. Buy empty capsules, which are available at many health food stores and pharmacies. Fill them with powdered turmeric, which can be purchased wherever culinary spices are sold.)

Lecithin   Lecithin is an excellent way to thin the bile and promote the flow of toxins out of the liver. Although made from soybeans, lecithin is permissible in the detox diet because it's refined so that the original, hard-to-digest proteins are no longer present. It has demonstrated an ability to significantly improve the solubility of bile. We use it in our clinic for all gallbladder diseases and feel that it's also helpful in liver diseases.

One study found that lecithin was able to delay the onset of—and even reverse—cirrhosis of the liver. In this study, lecithin actually prevented liver scarring induced by alcohol damage. This is remarkable because it shows that lecithin can both improve bile flow and protect the liver. It can also be used to treat high cholesterol and hepatitis. However, more is not necessarily better when it comes to bile lubricants. In fact, stimulating bile flow too quickly can cause headaches and gallbladder pain.

The recommended dosage of lecithin is 500 mg three times daily.

Strategy Group Four: Bile Binding

After the bile "shoots" through the liver and biliary (bile) system, it squirts out into the intestines. Unless something is there to bind the bile, "packaging" it for excretion, certain toxic compounds that it contains can be reabsorbed through the highly permeable membranes of the intestinal tract. Because detoxification aims to enhance the removal of all this toxic bile, charcoal should be used to bind it in the intestines. Soluble fiber from vegetables and whole grains will also help bind the bile. The bowels must move easily and regularly to prevent toxic bile from remaining in contact with the membranes of the large intestine any longer than is necessary.

Charcoal   In the intestines, toxins processed in the liver and excreted in the bile fluid mix with bacteria. Some of these bacteria produce an enzyme called beta-glucuronidase, which releases the toxins from the bile, allowing them to be reabsorbed and circulated through the body again. However, once bile is bound with charcoal, the toxins it carries can't be detached, even when washed with blood plasma or gastric fluids.

Charcoal acts like a sponge, and it has a tremendous absorptive capacity relative to its size. For example, 1 quart of pulverized charcoal can absorb 80 quarts of ammonia. Activated charcoal can absorb bacteria, viruses, bacterial toxins, and even hormones. It has been used for Asiatic cholera, dysentery, diarrhea, and dyspepsia. Charcoal is especially useful in conditions of harmful bacteria in the intestines. Even patients with liver failure can benefit from large doses of charcoal because it effectively prevents the buildup of toxins in the blood. Charcoal's ability to act as an antidote to poison has been known for more than a hundred years, and it's still used in hospitals today as the treatment of choice for certain types of poisoning.

Charcoal holds on to toxins more effectively than any other substance. It's safe, effective, and inexpensive. Wood charcoal, the only type that's recommended, is available as a supplement in capsule form.

The recommended dosage of charcoal is 2 capsules per meal or up to 2 teaspoons in powdered form. For best results, take it on an empty stomach. For those using charcoal in their seven-day program, I usually recommend it only to those patients who have severe digestive problems. Those who have a lot of acid, mucus in the stool, flatulence, and abdominal pain (irritable bowel syndrome) are the ones who get the most benefit.

Soluble Fiber   Fiber is essential for detoxification in the intestines. The longer food stays in the intestines, the more likely it is to putrefy and create poisons that leak into the bloodstream. An adequate amount of soluble fiber prevents constipation by providing the bulk that allows digested food to move through the bowel easily. Fiber decreases the overgrowth of endotoxin-producing bacteria, shortens the time that toxins stay in the intestines, and reduces toxin absorption. It increases the excretion of bacterial toxins and protein putrefaction products found in the intestines.

The recommended dosage of soluble fiber is found in the EcoTox diet of rice, fresh fruits and vegetables, and a rice protein concentrate.

Strategy Group Five: Replacing Bacteria

As we discussed in chapter 4, there are at least four hundred microorganisms in the human gastrointestinal tract, some of which are helpful and others that aren't. These "good" and "bad" bacteria compete for space and nutrients. "Friendly" bacteria, also called probiotics, secrete substances to kill the harmful, pathogenic microbes that inhabit the intestinal tract and breed there when conditions are favorable. If the balance between the two is disrupted, the population of hostile intestinal bacteria grows abnormally large, allowing bacterial poisons to enter the bloodstream. Altered intestinal bacteria and/or bowel toxemia (the presence of toxins produced by bacteria in the bowel) have been implicated in a wide range of disease conditions, from rheumatoid arthritis and ankylosing spondylitis to colitis, diabetes, meningitis, myasthenia gravis, thyroid disease, and bowel cancer.

Antibiotics, steroids, and birth control pills commonly upset the normal bacterial equilibrium in the intestines. Poor diet and chronic constipation are also contributing factors. Reseeding the intestines with favorable bacteria, taken orally as a nutritional supplement, creates an optimum, balanced environment, protecting the intestines and the rest of the body from dangerous bacterial insurgents.

The most commonly recommended sources of favorable bacteria are *Lactobacillus acidophilus* and the *L. bifidus* strains. *Lactobacillus* bacteria are normally found in the large and small intestines and vaginal lining. To inhibit the growth of other less favorable bacteria, *Lactobacillus* must be present in extremely high quantities.

Some doctors are beginning to consider the yeast *Saccharomyces boulardii* as another therapeutic probiotic agent for intestinal disorders. It has been used extensively in Europe with good results and is beginning to gain acceptance in the United States. It has been shown to soothe mucous membranes and is very good for patients with chronic intestinal irritation.

Whey concentrates, a special milk immunoglobulin made from cow's milk, are another form of probiotics that many doctors recommend. Whey concentrates contain secretory IgA, an immunoglobulin that protects your intestines by binding with harmful bacteria. This makes it more difficult for the bacteria to adhere to the intestinal wall so that they do less damage.

Supplementation with probiotics is especially important in a number of situations: after taking a course of antibiotic therapy (this also applies to nursing infants whose mothers are on antibiotic medication), when using birth control pills or steroids, and in cases of chronic constipation, monilial (yeast) and bacterial vaginitis, and gastrointestinal infections or inflammation. It is also highly beneficial for those who are lactose intolerant; who have high serum cholesterol, chronic liver disease, oral infections with herpes simplex, or cancer; and who experience diarrhea from radiation or bacterial or viral infections. It can also be used as a preventive against diarrhea in infants and in the control of acne.

In adults, a dose of 15 to 20 billion organisms per day is helpful in cases of acute bacterial or yeast infections.

The recommended dosage of supplemental probiotics is 3 to 7 billion organisms daily for extended use as well as during the week of detoxification. The ideal forms of supplementation are *L. acidophilus* and *L. bifidus*, in capsules or as a liquid, which are usually available from a health food store. Quality products containing live viable bacterial cultures require refrigeration and are best taken between meals. (Supplementation from fermented products, such as yogurt, is not recommended because doses aren't standardized and the cultures are likely no longer alive.)

Because of the tremendous amount of medical research documenting its effectiveness, we recommend the use of *acidophilus* in our program. Health care practitioners are increasingly using other probiotics as well, such as *S. boulardii* and whey concentrates, so we include suggested dosages for your information. The recommended dosage of *S. boulardii* is 300 mg three times a day.

The recommended dosage of whey concentrates is 1 teaspoon dissolved in warm water three times daily.

Strategy Group Six: Decreasing Intestinal Permeability

The walls of the intestines are designed to allow only very small molecules to pass through them. If the walls become more permeable, compounds meant to be excreted from the bowel leak into the bloodstream. When this leakage occurs, a kind of biological Alamo is created: Toxic enemies invade the stronghold of our bodies, our resistance weakens, and eventually we're overrun and defeated. The amino acid glutamine, gamma oryzanol found in rice products, vitamin E, pantothenic acid, zinc, soluble fiber, and inulin from Jerusalem artichokes have been shown to heal damaged intestinal membranes.

Glutamine   The amino acid glutamine is a fuel burned by intestinal cells and is essential for their proper function. It increases the thickness of the membranes in the intestines so that the wrong molecules can't pass through and circulate in the blood. It prevents the movement of bacteria across the intestinal membranes, increases the secretion of valuable immune antibodies in the intestinal membranes, and generally improves the health of intestinal immune function.

At our clinic, we saw a young boy who had been given antibiotics just after he was born. Ever since that time, he had terrible eczema, which was treated with all types of topical creams. When he finally came to us, he was four years old. We immediately started a program to treat his intestinal permeability and had excellent results. The program included doses of glutamine three times daily.

The recommended dosage of glutamine is 500 mg three times daily.

Strategy Group Seven: Vitamins, Minerals, and Nutrients

Nutrients are integral to the formation and action of all biochemical processes in the body. Detoxification biochemistry requires specific vitamin and mineral support. In fact, many of the benefits ascribed to vitamin therapy are linked to their participation in the cycle of detoxification. We have included a few common vitamins, minerals, and other nutritional substances that are important in detoxification.

Bioflavonoids   Bioflavonoids, which include more than six thousand different food-based substances, have a natural antioxidant, tissue-protective capacity. Vitamin C replenishes the antioxidant capability of bioflavonoids, so the two are best used in combination. The bioflavonoids we suggest for detoxification are catechin, silymarin, and curcumin.

Catechin is found in green tea. Green tea contains several polyphenol catechins (a type of antioxidant bioflavonoid), but the strongest is EGCG, which was found to have two hundred times more antioxidant strength than vitamin E in protecting cell membranes. Studies have shown that drinking green tea (as distinct from black tea) offers smokers some protection from cardiovascular disease. Its ability to activate detoxification enzymes in the liver has also been shown to provide a defense against cancer. Catechin has a special affinity for the liver, so it can be used effectively in the treatment of liver diseases, hepatitis, and alcohol-related liver syndromes. It also offers protection from bacterial toxins in the intestines and from collagen diseases, such as rheumatoid arthritis and scleroderma, a condition in which the skin thickens and hardens.

Green tea does contain some caffeine, but is permissible because it's ideal for heavy coffee drinkers, mitigating the symptoms of caffeine withdrawal. It's safe and probably advised for those who feel a little sluggish and want a pick-me-up. It's also very good for people who need to lose weight.

The recommended dosage of catechins is at least 3 cups daily taken as green tea.

Silymarin   Silymarin, a substance comprised of a group of bioflavonoids found in milk thistle, can have very dramatic effects. Its antitoxin, antioxidant effects make it a substance for which there is no pharmaceutical replacement. No drug can protect your liver the way silymarin can because of its strong action against free radicals and its ability to enhance glutathione production by more than 35 percent, thus increasing liver detoxification. Its effectiveness has been measured by lower enzyme markers on liver function tests, which reflect nonspecific liver cell inflammation. Its low cost, safety, and effectiveness place it at the top of all natural products.

Silymarin is truly a wonder plant and has been used successfully in the treatment of the following:

- Neurological complications caused by diabetes
- Fatty liver disease in diabetic patients
- Nausea caused by high levels of hormones naturally produced during pregnancy
- Chronic alcoholic liver diseases
- Toxic exposure to industrial chemicals
- Acute viral hepatitis
- Cirrhosis of the liver
- Immune system and liver protection

The recommended dosage of silymarin is 200 mg three times daily.

Vitamin A We recommend vitamin A—not beta-carotene but rather retinol or retinoic acid—for many types of immune and toxic diseases. Studies have shown that exposure to environmental toxins increases the body's need for vitamin A.

The recommended dosage of vitamin A is 10,000 to 30,000 IU daily. Doses over 10,000 IU per day need to be on a doctor's recommendation.

Riboflavin (Vitamin B₂)   Riboflavin is important in the production of energy in the cells and is also involved in the production of the critical detoxifying antioxidant glutathione. Low levels of riboflavin diminish glutathione's antioxidant defense. Using riboflavin may turn your urine yellow.

The recommended dosage of riboflavin is 10 to 20 mg daily.

Niacin (Vitamin B₃)   Niacin has been used to treat high cholesterol, diabetes, schizophrenia, and cerebrovascular insufficiency (poor blood flow to the brain). It plays a critical role in energy metabolism in the cell and in producing the neurotransmitters that are necessary for normal brain functioning. It is also involved in detoxification reactions.

The recommended dosage of niacin is 10 to 1,000 mg daily. If you're taking more than 1,000 mg daily, ask your doctor to perform liver tests to monitor your progress: In rare cases, individuals are sensitive to high levels of niacin, and instead of helping the liver, niacin can cause liver inflammation in them.

Pantothenic Acid   At our clinic, we call pantothenic acid the "stress vitamin" because of the many ways that it protects the body. Pantothenic acid is important for the synthesis of coenzyme A and glucuronic acid, both of which the body uses in detoxification of drugs and toxins. Coenzyme A also helps to burn sugars and fats to release energy in the form of ATP and aids in the synthesis of fatty acids, cholesterol, steroids, phospholipids, and porphyrin. It supports the synthesis of the neurotransmitter acetylcholine and helps repair damaged tissue. Pantothenic acid can control antioxidant enzymes, which modulate cellular free-radical reactions, and support and improve white blood cell activity for healing wounds. It's an important nutrient in times of increased biochemical demand due to injury and toxin exposure.

The recommended dosage of pantothenic acid is 500 mg daily.

Cobalamin (Vitamin B$_{12}$), Folic Acid, and Pyridoxine (Vitamin B$_6$) Because of its ability to donate a part of itself as a methyl group, vitamin B$_{12}$ can help detoxify the amino acid homocysteine. Folic acid, vitamin B$_6$, and betaine are also able to detoxify excess homocysteine from a high-protein diet. Because these three vitamins are interconnected in this chemical reaction, all of them should be included in an ongoing supplementation program, especially for those who eat meat regularly.

Vitamin B$_{12}$ can also help those who are sensitive to sulfites, which are used as a preservative in salad bar foods and wines. Asthma-like symptoms, especially after eating foods that contain sulfites, are a sign of sulfite sensitivity. In this situation, vitamin B$_{12}$ should be used in combination with molybdenum supplementation, 100 to 600 mcg per day.

The recommended dosage of vitamin B$_{12}$ is 1,000 mcg daily.

Magnesium, Copper, Manganese, Zinc, Molybdenum, and Selenium Enzymes that manage detoxification in the cells need all these minerals to become active. The minerals become reaction sites for enzyme action. Without these minerals, enzymes can't do their jobs. Mineral deficiency is usually caused by vegetarian and weight-loss diets, alcoholism, old age, or protein deficiency.

Magnesium is the number-one mineral deficiency we see in our clinic. Such deficiencies are so common that we put all our patients on magnesium supplementation. The mineral is used in the treatment of asthma, cardiovascular diseases, diabetes, fatigue, fibromyalgia, migraine headaches, and PMS. The body uses it in more than three hundred enzyme reactions, generating energy and driving the detoxification machinery of enzymes.

Copper, manganese, and zinc are important in the formation of the antioxidant enzyme superoxide dismutase. Zinc works with many other enzymes and is important to the structure of cell membranes. It's also an essential component of hormones and stimulates healing by nourishing nutrient-hungry cells in the process of replicating. Extreme zinc deficiency manifests as lesions in the skin and intestinal tract. Diets limited in animal protein, the richest source of zinc, pose the highest risk for zinc deficiency.

Molybdenum deficiencies can lead to sulfite toxicity because the enzyme that breaks down sulfite, sulfite oxidase, depends on molybdenum. This deficiency also causes asthma and even neurological damage. Xanthine oxidase, which reacts with molecules used to construct DNA, is another enzyme that requires adequate levels of molybdenum.

Selenium is used to form the enzyme glutathione peroxidase, which protects against free-radical damage. It also protects against heavy metals, such as lead, mercury, aluminum, and cadmium.

The recommended dosages of these minerals are as follows:

- Zinc: 15 mg daily

- Copper: 2 mg daily

- Magnesium: 500 mg daily

- Manganese: 30 mg daily (as recommended for the seven-day detoxification program; 10 mg daily is appropriate for maintenance care) (This should only be maintained under a doctor's supervision.)

- Molybdenum: 0.5 mg daily

- Selenium: 0.2 mg daily

Strategy Group Eight: Cathartics (As Needed)

The intestines are the most active site of immune function in our body. Cathartics have a laxative effect that purges the bowels, purifying and emptying them. Because this action encourages optimum immune response, cathartics are powerful agents for treating acute health problems. Removing irritants and cleansing the bowel improves immune recognition, the ability of disease-fighting molecules to recognize disease-causing invaders. That's why it's said that the doctor or patient who heals the bowels controls the immune system and thus controls disease.

The herbs listed as cathartics are for use only in cases of constipation or fever and for those who are in a severe toxic state, symptoms of which are a heavily coated tongue, bad breath, offensive body odor, excessive intestinal gas, irritability, and poor appetite. If you develop a fever during your detoxification week, consult with a health care practitioner to be sure that it's the result of the cleansing process and not some other cause.

O. G. Carroll, a well-known naturopathic doctor of the post-Depression era, used cathartic herbs to help in the early stages of many types of acute disease, especially in cases of acute infection or inflammation. According to Dr. Carroll, colds could be aborted if you took this formula and skipped the next two meals. He used the same herbal combination that we recommend to treat the early stages of many types of acute disease, including poor digestion, roundworms, pinworms, angina, and asthma.

A basic cathartic formula consists of 4 parts of wormwood (*Artemesia absinthum*) and 2 parts of cape aloe (*Aloe socotrina*), together in capsule form. Wormwood acts as a tonic for the upper portion of the intestinal tract, and cape aloe stimulates the lower intestine. We consider this herbal formula a frontline treatment in any healing crisis.

The recommended dosage of this cathartic is 1 capsule daily as strong laxative action or 2 capsules every four hours until the bowels move. Cathartics should not be taken for nausea unless the nausea is caused by food poisoning.

Strategy Group Nine: Antiparasitics (As Needed)

Much consumer literature has been published attributing the cause of many chronic diseases to the presence of parasites.

What Is a Healing Crisis

A healing crisis is a change in health during detoxification that is characterized by fever, diarrhea, headaches, loss of appetite, and other symptoms common to acute infections. Because it can be difficult to determine the difference between an illness and a healing crisis, when symptoms appear it is best to consult with a health care professional, preferably one who is trained in detoxification medicine.

Intestinal worms and microorganisms, such as *Giardia* and *Blastocystis hominus,* have been cited as the source of much human suffering, from cancer to AIDS. Both the curious and the desperate are using formulations containing cloves and black walnut hulls, both of which are folk remedies for parasites, in the hopes that this diagnosis is accurate.

If you have chronic disease symptoms and suspect parasites, see your doctor and request laboratory testing for parasites. If the results are positive, proceed with an appropriate treatment. Certain herbs and extracts have been found to be effective for parasites, but for some types of infestation, drug therapies might be warranted. We don't recommend a cleansing for parasites unless you know that you have a parasite problem.

Clearing intestinal parasites from your system involves treatments for worms, amoebas, and yeast. Each of these is a significant subject in itself, and it's beyond the scope of this book to include a complete review of all varieties of parasite therapy. We have listed some antiparasitic herbs and included some treatment recommendations for each parasite group. However, this list in no way represents the only available therapy protocols. *Warning:* These herb therapies may not be appropriate for pregnant woman. Please consult your physician.

Worms: Wormwood (*Artemesia absinthum*) Wormwood is a type of sage and a member of the daisy family. Absinthol, the volatile oil the plant contains, makes its taste extremely bitter. This oil is remarkably effective against worms. Historically, wormwood was used in the production of bitters, an after-dinner digestive drink popular in Europe.

Unfortunately, in producing the drink, toxic substances in the plant were concentrated to such a degree that, when ingested over long periods of time, it led to neurological problems. Today, wormwood preparations, in the form of tea or a powder-containing capsule, contain negligible amounts of the toxic elements, so there's no risk of dangerous side effects unless taken in doses exceeding the recommended amount. In addition to its antiparasitic properties, wormwood is a very effective medicine for liver and gallbladder diseases.

The recommended dosage of wormwood is 1 teaspoon in a glass of boiling water, steeped for ten minutes, taken in 3 doses for one or two days. The recommended dose for capsules is 2 capsules per dose.

Amoebas: Papain Some of our patients who travel extensively in South America and other tropical countries have mentioned that papaya fasts are used in these countries for amoeba infestations. In our clinic, we use papain, an enzyme from papaya that has the ability to dissolve parasites in the intestines. We have achieved very good results using papain in pill form. The treatment is safe and relatively inexpensive.

The recommended dosage of papain is 1 tablet three times daily between meals for one week while using the Eco-Tox program. Stop taking papain if you have any abdominal discomfort or irritation.

Yeast Overgrowth: Undecylcenic Acid It is not well known that undecyclenic acid, the fatty acid in castor oil, is very effective against intestinal yeast overgrowth. Many effective antifungals are available as pharmaceutical drugs and natural antifungal agents, and we can't say for sure whether undecyclenic acid is better than any other antifungal. However, we can say that our patients have had favorable results with this treatment.

The recommended dosage of undecylcenic acid is 2 tablets three times daily between meals.

Tips for Supplementation

Because massive amounts of toxins flood into the system during the first two days of fasting, the body needs antioxidants, which tend to prevent headaches and feelings of sickness. You can use a full supplemental program during your fast, but if vitamins and other nutrient supplements make you queasy when you take them on an empty stomach, you can use the following three critical nutrients alone: charcoal, 1 capsule three times daily; vitamin C, 500 mg three times daily; and milk thistle, 1 capsule three times daily.

We have found—after using pharmaceutical-grade essential oils orally, under the tongue, on hundreds of patients—that this an effective method to stimulate rapid liver detoxification, although there is no medical literature to support this recommendation. If you can find oral-grade essential oils, we highly recommend it. We use a combination of ginger, chamomile, and rosemary, 1 drop of each, once a day for seven days.

Your baseline supplementation plan should include the following:

- A good-quality multivitamin that contains at least the recommended daily allowances of vitamins A, B-complex, and E plus 15 mg zinc, 2 mg copper, 30 mg manganese, 0.5 mg molybdenum, 0.2 mg selenium, and 500 mg magnesium
- Vitamin C
- Milk thistle
- *Lactobacillus acidophilus*

If you have a specific condition that you want to address, add those supplements that apply to you. Those who are diagnosed with parasites, for example, need an antiparasitic. Those who are chronically constipated benefit by including a cathartic. If you have a history of chronic liver inflammation, you might want to include lipoic acid or glycine. If you have a history of bowel inflammation or food allergies or have other reasons to suspect that you have intestinal permeability, add glutamine to your list.

Remember that different people have different levels of tolerance for specific vitamins. Be aware that your body might not react well to larger-than-normal doses of certain vitamins. Some of our patients have reactions to vitamin C, some to niacin, and some to B vitamins. In these cases, we search for alternative choices to achieve the same effect.

To help you select the correct supplementation program for you, use the following guidelines:

1. If you have liver disease or a chronic illness such as fibromyalgia or chronic fatigue syndrome, get a liver detoxification profile (see chapter 7). Some of our toxic patients show abnormal values on this test. When this happens, we need to determine the cause of the abnormality. Some of the causes are alcohol and/or drug use, pesticide exposure, or intestinal endotoxins. A precise analysis provides the information necessary to correct the problem and stimulate proper Phase 1 and Phase 2 detoxification.

2. Provide adequate antioxidant support for oxidative stress, as determined by your lifestyle, occupation, and/or lab testing. Oxidative stress testing is done with a blood test (see chapter 7) or through a thorough evaluation by a trained health care practitioner.

3. Intestinal permeability impairs or depletes nutrient-dependent detoxification. If you have high intestinal permeability, you'll need to follow a more nutrient-dense program than someone who has low intestinal permeability. To see

whether you might need a lab evaluation, see the discussion of intestinal permeability in chapter 4.

4. Some people metabolize nutrients and toxins differently than others. You might need to experiment with higher or lower doses of a supplement to achieve the best results. Blood tests can check for healthy levels of amino acids, fats, minerals, and vitamins (see chapter 7) and point to any imbalances and deficiencies you might have.

5. Pharmaceutical drugs alter your body's detoxification capability. For example, selective serotonin reuptake inhibitors (SSRIs), such as Prozac, inhibit liver detoxification enzymes. If you're on such medication, you should be evaluated by a qualified professional to determine which supplements to use, depending on your individual needs.

6. Repeated antibiotic use and chronic bowel inflammation need special attention. This problem can take months to solve and will not necessarily disappear in one week. We have seen patients with excess bacterial toxins in the intestinal tract suffer from impaired liver detoxification. These patients are usually given higher doses of detoxification nutrients. If you have a history of repeated antibiotic use or currently have a diagnosis of bowel inflammation, you should suspect that bacterial toxicity in the intestines is a problem for you. Treat the problem and prevent its recurrence by following the instructions in this book for seven-day detoxification three or four times a year. It can take several weeks, spread over months of this program, to rebuild a damaged bowel.

Module Three: Circulation Therapy

It's essential to tune your piano or your car's engine if they are to work properly. Your body and mind are no different. This module is devoted to tuning your body by establishing proper circulation of the blood and lymphatic fluids. This is especially important while you're undergoing a seven-day detoxification program. In addition to following a specialized diet and taking nutritional supplements, we recommend four simple methods to increase blood circulation and metabolic rate: hydrotherapy, dry skin brushing, exercise therapy, and breath and mind training. These methods also release tension to facilitate the removal of toxins from the body.

The circulatory system is very important for all your organs, tissues, and cells. It carries waste products away so that they can be eliminated. Hydrotherapy improves blood flow to vital organs and reduces fat in the tissues. Exercise therapy can increase the metabolic rate and mechanically push body fluids through the filtering organs of the lymph system. Breath and mind training aim to reduce tension in the nervous system that disturbs the delicate enzyme systems in the liver, making it more difficult for toxins to be released and removed.

Hydrotherapy

A simple, traditional health care method, such as hydrotherapy, is rooted in common sense. It has the added value of being time tested. It can be done without medical assistance or specialized knowledge. Years of clinical observation and experience of doctors skilled in detoxification medicine confirm the effectiveness of this therapy. It has been the cornerstone of traditional naturopathic methods of detoxification therapy in both North America and Europe for 150 years. *Rational Hydrotherapy*, a 1,200-page book by John Harvey Kellogg, M.D., published in 1923, describes 224 ways to apply hydrotherapy.

Hydrotherapy consists of using hot and cold water in different ways to increase the flow of blood to various tissues of the body, especially the skin. You must do one type of hydrotherapy each day. This aspect of your detoxification program is very important because it regulates circulation in organs that are under stress during detoxification, healing illness and preventing disease. We have chosen four of the easiest methods for you to apply, listed in order of simplicity.

A word of caution: If you go outside after any hydrotherapy treatment and get chilled because your hair is wet or you are not warmly dressed, you can get very sick (severe bronchitis and pneumonia are two possibilities). Always stay warm after the treatment and make sure that you are thoroughly covered and dry. Also, it's best to do hydrotherapy on an empty stomach. Ideal times are first thing in the morning and last thing at night. No food should be consumed following dinner in the early evening. These are also good times for exercise and meditation.

Shower Method   Take a hot shower for five minutes, allowing the water to run on your back. The water should be as hot as you can tolerate. Then switch the water to pure cold and leave it running while you count thirty breaths (fast ones). Follow this with another five minutes of hot water, taking care not to burn yourself, and then cold water again for thirty breaths. Repeat this hot-cold cycle one more time. After you've finished three rounds, get out of the shower and dry off quickly. Get into bed and lie under the covers for thirty minutes, making sure you stay extremely warm. Then get up and continue your day.

Bed rest is important because it allows circulation, which has been opened up, to continue for a brief period of time. As soon as you begin to move around or get excited by activity or thoughts, the blood flow to the abdomen becomes restricted again. Because the main idea is to get blood flowing to the intestines, the best results are achieved when the stomach is empty (digestion requires blood circulation to the stomach).

This therapy relaxes the tension of the sympathetic nervous system and increases blood flow through the filtering organs of the abdominal and chest region. The alternating hot and cold water on the back stimulates the sympathetic nerve chain that runs up and down the spine on both sides. When done correctly, you should experience a cool feeling in your abdomen from the increased blood flow and have a sensation of being clean inside and out.

If you don't have time to get under the covers, make sure that you're warmly dressed after the shower. This hot and cold showering can be done twice a day but must be done at least once a day.

Bath and Wet Sheet Method   This can be done instead of or in addition to the shower method. Fill a bathtub with water that is as hot as you can tolerate (usually about 107 degrees Fahrenheit) and lie in it for fifteen to forty-five minutes, until you can't stand the heat any longer. Get out of the bath and wrap yourself in a cold, wet sheet.

Chill the sheet in the refrigerator or the freezer. To prepare the sheet, soak it in cold water, wring it out well, and put it in a plastic bag in your refrigerator a few hours prior to bathing. You want the wet sheet to be as cold as possible. If you chill the sheet in the freezer, be sure not to leave it there more than an hour, or it will become stiff and difficult to handle. If your kitchen and bathroom are relatively far apart, you can either ask a helper to bring it to you when you are ready or keep it in a small picnic cooler in the bathroom.

Wrapped in this sheet, get into a bed lined with towels and pile layers of blankets on top of yourself. You'll be chilled for a minute or so, then you'll become warm, and finally you'll become very hot and start sweating. Stay under the blankets for thirty to sixty minutes; you might even fall asleep.

We suggest doing this treatment before bed. When you get up after your hour of sweating, quickly change into warm pajamas, remove the wet towels from the bed (making sure that all your bedding is dry), and go to sleep for the night. If you do this at any other time, make sure that you dry off thoroughly and dress warmly before going out. It's very easy to get chilled after this treatment, so be extra careful. The chill will upset the flow of blood into the skin and could cause a respiratory infection.

The wet sheet and bath method is especially good for the skin and lymphatic system. It can also create a healing crisis (an immune reaction brought on by detoxification) accompanied by a low fever; this is especially good for toxic conditions. Wet sheet treatments are very beneficial at the beginning stages of a cold, when there is a feeling of chill with a slight sore throat.

Constitutional Hydrotherapy   Dr. Bastyr, the famous naturopathic physician for whom Bastyr University in Seattle, Washington, is named, was emphatic about the importance of using constitutional hydrotherapy for people suffering from chronic diseases. It works by intensifying blood circulation to the kidneys, intestines, and liver. This promotes filtering by the liver and kidneys as well as better digestion of food, boosting nutrition to the cells of vital organs and tissues. It enhances oxygenation and circulation of blood and lymph, toxin elimination, and immune system activity, thereby strengthening the body. It's a difficult treatment to do alone, so you'll likely need a helper.

To begin, prepare two sets of towels. One set of two bath-sized towels should be soaked in hot water and wrung out, and the other set should be soaked in cold water and wrung out. Lie on your back, bare from the neck to the waist. Your helper layers the hot damp towels on top of you from the collarbone to the pubic bone and then covers you up to the neck with warm blankets. After ten minutes, the hot towels are replaced with cold ones, covering the same region of the body, and topped by warm blankets for ten minutes.

Repeat this procedure of alternating hot and cold towel packs, but instead lie on your stomach and have your helper apply packs to your back from the neck to the buttocks. For this treatment to work, it's essential that you keep the towel temperatures as hot and as cold as you can tolerate. Soaking the towels in cold water filled with ice cubes is a good idea. If you finish the treatment and the cold towels aren't warm from your body heat, replace them with a fresh set of hot towels, followed by another application of towels that are not quite so cold. End the treatment only when you are able to warm the cold towel packs with your own body heat, otherwise you will not derive any of its benefits.

Sauna Therapy   Saunas are extremely safe and have been used for thousands of years by many cultures. In the Ayurvedic medical tradition of India, sweating therapy is one of the five main methods for detoxification. Both the Finnish and various Native American peoples have long advocated the benefits of wet and dry heat to prompt intensive sweats. After each sauna session, you should take a cold shower to get the best results for circulation.

In chapter 4, we discussed that the skin acts like a second kidney. Our skin has an amazing 11,000 square feet of surface area, and our sweat is made of the fluids from the blood and lymph. When we sweat, some of the poisons these fluids contain are excreted through the skin.

We're convinced that the plan we've created offers the best of all solutions to a wide variety of health problems.

The wonderful thing about sauna therapy is that almost everyone seems to tolerate it well. Adults, healthy or ill, seem to benefit from saunas, except for patients with seizure disorders, who should not use this form of therapy.

Generally, sauna therapy is not recommended for children because they tend to dehydrate quickly. It's also not recommended for pregnant women or for those with a tendency to get headaches or get overheated easily. Nor should sauna therapy immediately follow intense exercise.

Research has shown that even patients who have heart disease and complex circulatory problems experience very few complications from saunas. Several studies have shown that sauna heat improves circulation and takes a load off the heart by relaxing constricted blood vessels and promoting better peripheral circulation.

Saunas are a powerful strategy for promoting detoxification through the skin.

The body stores many toxins in fatty tissue. Sweating therapy reduces fat stores quickly, releasing these poisons for excretion through the stimulation of receptors in the fat. Tissue biochemistry and nervous system functioning undergo changes in sauna therapy, activating fat stores and facilitating fat loss. As you sweat, a wide range of toxins that are stored in the fat and blood (e.g., PCBs, cadmium, lead, and industrial chemicals) are excreted through the skin. The heat of the sauna also encourages the body to burn fat stores quickly, and this effect continues as long as one remains in the sauna.

Scientific studies have been done to evaluate the effectiveness of sauna therapy for detoxification. In one study, fourteen firemen who were exposed to PCBs and subsequently developed neuropsychological problems six months after the fire underwent three weeks of a sauna program. They were compared with a "control" group of firemen from the same department who did not participate in the detoxification program. The control firemen showed significant impairment of memory for stories, visual images, and counting numbers backward. Conversely, retesting in the detoxification group showed significant improvement in scores in these three memory tests.

The technique of sweating therapy is simple. Use a low-temperature sauna, about 140 to 180 degrees Fahrenheit. Any sauna that you have access to is acceptable, including those at health and exercise clubs. Many hotels have saunas that can be used by non–hotel guests for a nominal fee. Sweating intensively, a person can lose as much as 3 liters (or about 8 pounds) of fluid per hour, so drink 1 quart of warm water before entering and take water into the sauna with you, continuing to drink throughout the length of your sweat. Begin by staying in the sauna for fifteen minutes, then come out for a cold-water rinse. Repeat this process for one hour. As you become more acclimated to the heat, increase your time every day until you reach two hours. The rinse therapy is important because it stimulates circulation in the skin and removes waste material being excreted through it.

Make sure that you're taking a mineral supplement during sauna treatments. Valuable minerals are lost in sweat and need to be replaced during detoxification treatment. Stop sauna therapy and consult a qualified professional if any problems arise, such as headaches, rashes, eye problems, or extreme dizziness and fatigue. If you find that the heat bothers your head, wrap a wet towel around it.

If sauna therapy is too difficult, try steam baths. You can get a steam bath installed in your shower or find companies that sell the type of steam box in which you sit with your head sticking out. Steam baths are easier to use because they make you sweat faster and aren't as dehydrating.

Dry Skin Brushing

Your skin does many things: It helps regulate body temperature, functions as an organ of both respiration and elimination, and participates in the absorption of oxygen and nutrients. The skin acts as a protective shield to the outside world. Surprisingly, although the skin weighs twice as much as the liver and brain, it receives only one-third the circulation.

Dry skin brushing is an old natural healing method used to increase blood and lymphatic circulation. (For more information about the lymphatic system and its important role in your health, see chapter 3.) Stimulating the skin improves circulation, a benefit for every organ of the body. Skin brushing removes dead skin cells, keeps the skin soft, improves blood and lymph circulation, helps control cellulite, and rids the body of toxins.

To use this method, brush your whole body once a day with a natural-bristle dry skin brush that you can find at health food stores. During your week of detoxification, do this after hydrotherapy. Your strokes should be short and brisk. Start with your arms, front and back, moving from the fingertips up into the armpit, always brushing toward the heart. Then do each leg, front and back, starting at the feet and brushing upward. Don't forget to brush the bottoms of the feet. Follow each leg up through the pelvis, buttocks, abdomen, and lower back. Then do the chest and upper back, always brushing toward the heart. If you want, you can lightly do the face and head, using downward strokes.

Keep the brush dry (never get it wet). Just as you wouldn't use someone else's toothbrush, be sure that only you use your skin brush. If skin brushing is painful, do it lightly and persevere—the discomfort will pass. Brush the whole body daily using at least one stroke for every section of skin. The chest, abdomen, and inner thigh should be done gently and carefully.

Exercise Therapy

Every cell of the body produces waste that must be metabolized and removed or the cell will die. Exercise is critical for health because it stimulates blood circulation and the movement of lymphatic fluid, making it easier for the body to eliminate these waste products. Exercise also promotes the reduction of fat reserves, a primary storage site for toxins. Mobilizing these fat reserves is a very important part of detoxification therapy.

Aerobic Exercise We feel that a little aerobic exercise every day is good for everyone, especially during detoxification. Such exercise can be bicycling, jogging, swimming, or brisk walking—anything that raises your heart rate for twenty minutes. Do this at least three times a week. People who are overweight or have knee and hip pain should try a low-impact aerobic exercise, such as swimming or walking on a treadmill. Exercise is optional on the fasting days; if you feel weak, don't push yourself.

Jumping rope is a good type of aerobic exercise. It's easy, can be done at home, and offers a good workout that will increase aerobic capacity, timing, and coordination. It's excellent for the calves, hips, thighs, and abdominal muscles.

If you're in good aerobic shape, start with 200 skips per session and work up to 1,000. Jumping should be crisp, without any errors. If you can't manage 200 skips, do as many as you can to start with, adding another ten each day. When you make a mistake, pause and then resume counting from where you left off. Rest briefly and catch your breath as often as you need to. If you're diligent in practice, you'll see improvement over time.

Mind Training

Detoxification includes the mind. A negative, tension-filled mind does not support well-being. Although the main focus of the EcoTox program is the biochemical purification of the blood, our clinical experience has shown the value of a program that addresses each person's mental state. Internal tension is a result of stress. This tension causes toxicity and eventually disease.

The body reacts to stress by secreting hormones that disturb the detoxification mechanisms. Thousands of years ago, physicians in China noted that emotional disturbances such as anger upset the liver's ability to function. Herbs, acupuncture, and qi gong exercises were often recommended for the problem of tension irritating the liver.

Working with breathing is an effective way to calm the mind. It affects the involuntary control centers in the brain that issue stress and alarm signals to the rest of the body. There is a wealth of current medical literature supporting the benefits of breath training. Breathing exercises have strong, measurable effects on the body. As these exercises relax the mind, they help to oxygenate the blood and, most important, regulate the autonomic nervous system. Current research has affirmed the powerful effect that these exercises have on asthma, diabetes, chronic gastrointestinal disorders, and psychosomatic and psychiatric dysfunction.

It's easy to see the effect of mental states on your breathing patterns. When you're agitated, your breathing is agitated. When you're angry, your breaths are short and uneven. Conversely, when you're in a peaceful, relaxed state, the breath is long, fine, and barely perceptible. The following breathing exercise offers a simple way to start relieving mental stress.

Alternate-Nostril Breathing   Sit in a chair with your spine straight or on the floor with a cushion under the hips. Gently exhale all the air from your lungs. Close the right nostril by pressing with the thumb of the right hand. Inhale slowly and deeply through the left nostril until the lungs are full. With the lungs full, remove your thumb from the right side of your nose and press the left nostril closed with your ring finger and exhale through the right nostril. Inhale through the right nostril, slowly and deeply. When the lungs are full again, close the right nostril with your thumb as before and exhale through the left nostril. This completes one round. Begin with ten rounds and gradually increase to thirty.

The autonomic nervous system regulates the involuntary action of the intestines, heart, and hormone glands. It's divided into two parts: the sympathetic nervous system and the parasympathetic nervous system. Both are affected by stress. The sympathetic nervous system is turned on during stress and causes increased heart rate and elevated blood pressure. Alternate-nostril breathing has been shown to decrease sympathetic nervous system tone, altering the stress response, and cause shifts in hemispherical electrical activity in the brain.

After you've acquired the skill of breathing in this way, combine timed breathing with alternate-nostril breathing. Count to ten slowly while inhaling, and then count to ten slowly while exhaling. When you can do this comfortably, increase the count to fifteen. When you can inhale and exhale slowly to a count of twenty, change the pattern by exhaling for twice as long as you inhale. Start with an inhalation of fifteen counts and an exhalation of thirty counts. Work up to an inhalation of twenty-five counts and an exhalation of fifty. If you get to this point and want to learn more, contact a qualified yoga teacher for further information.

Follow your breathing exercise with a mental exercise meant to help you relax deeply and increase your self-awareness. Concentrate on experiencing the present while ignoring thoughts of the past and future, reflecting on your own state in a calm, natural, intentional way. The best results are achieved when this is done every day. Some religious, spiritual, and psychological systems refer to this type of mental exercise or mind training as meditation, prayer, awareness, affirmations, or relaxation therapy.

There's no mystical mumbo-jumbo and no trances—just an effort to make the mind as clear and quiet as it can possibly be. When you do this as described here, you should gradually feel your body relax as well; tension in the facial muscles is released and a mood-enhancing blood flow to the brain occurs. You might also notice a slowing of the heart rate and a change in negative emotional states.

Calming the Mind   Because thoughts are what make up the mind, emptying the mind of all thoughts gives us an opportunity to achieve a calm, peaceful state of mind. If we can practice achieving this on a daily basis, it becomes a habit. A habit of inner peace is the beginning of a healthy mind.

To begin, sit in a relaxed position with your back straight and your eyes gently focused on the floor in front of you. Sense your breath as it enters your nostrils, and mentally follow it as it fills your lungs and empties from your chest as you exhale. Count each breath (as 1, 2, 3, 4, 5, and so on) without allowing thoughts to interfere. Every time a thought interferes, go back to counting from the number 1. Try counting up to 100 without your mind being disturbed by thoughts.

Do this for ten minutes.

Shavasana: A Relaxing Yoga Posture   Take five minutes to relax your body and mind with shavasana (the corpse pose) after you exercise and before you go to bed. The corpse pose looks like a sleeping position to anyone viewing it, but it's quite different because it's done with consciousness and awareness. If performed correctly before bed, the amount of sleep needed can be reduced and the sleep that you get is much more refreshing.

To begin, lie on your back with palms on the bed or floor facing up. Inhale deeply and exhale through your nose. With each exhalation, visualize all your tension leaving your body. Each exhalation should accomplish this more effectively than the previous one. Sense your body and your hands, feet, abdomen, throat, and eyes getting heavier and heavier as you exhale tension out of your body. Do this for fifty breaths.

Yoga   The benefits of yoga for detoxification are unequaled. In our experience, people who practice yoga regularly are by far the healthiest of all our patients. Our personal experience confirms that yoga training is ideal for attaining optimal health. Yoga encourages the proper circulation of blood and lymph fluid, enhances digestion, reduces nervous tension, strengthens the endocrine system, lubricates the joints, reduces excess fat, improves concentration, and provides resistance to hunger and to the extremes of heat and cold. Every organ system in the body benefits from yoga. To add the practice of yoga to your lifestyle, follow these rules:

- Find a trained, qualified teacher to help you.
- Avoid teachers who emphasize their own personal talents.
- Be strict: Do the exercises regularly and at the same time every day.
- Be sure that the stomach is empty; four hours after eating is the best time to begin.
- Make sure there's no draft or wind where you're exercising.
- Lie down for a short period of time after exercising.

Most doctors recognize that any treatment program will fail if negative mental and emotional states continue to dominate. Nurturing positive intentions and feelings of love, joy, compassion, and even-mindedness toward all situations should be a part every health care plan. Daily relaxation is a powerful medicine that allows your body to heal.

The only way to avoid mental and emotional pain is to cultivate selfless, humble, and altruistic qualities. Affirmations, self-hypnosis, psychological counseling, dream journals, prayer, and meditation cleanse and heal the nonphysical dimensions of health. Positive emotional states of joy, compassion, pure love, and religious devotion remove the painful presence of negative mental and emotional states of mind. Highly evolved positive emotional states manifest as feelings of oneness with creation and a unity with the entire world.

A Sample Daily Training Schedule for Module Three

7 A.M.: Exercise, breath training, mind training, hydrotherapy, dry brushing

10 A.M.: Stretch

5 P.M.: Exercise/yoga, sauna, hydrotherapy, dry brushing

10 P.M.: Shavasana

Summary: Seven-Day Detox Program Guidelines

- Drink at least 2 quarts of water daily.
- Dilute fresh and bottled fruit juice with 50 percent water.
- Use only pure spring, distilled, or filtered water.
- Use only organically grown produce.
- Take all nutritional supplements with meals (unless indicated otherwise).
- Drink a rice protein shake twice daily as a snack between meals.
- Eat beets daily when not fasting.
- Get at least one hour of exercise daily.
- Sweat every day.

- Sleep at least six to seven hours a night.
- Avoid eating if you're not hungry.
- Avoid caffeinated beverages.
- Avoid activities at night that tend to be exciting, stimulating, or enervating (energy depleting) such as watching television or going to the theater, movies, or parties. Take this week to rest your mind as well as your body.
- Avoid products with sugar or preservatives added (read all labels).

Things to Do

To get yourself on the path to good health, write the following down on a paper and make an "action list" to get started.

1. Hair analysis: We recommend everyone have a hair analysis. It is quick and easy to do, and the information is very reliable and useful. Some labs provide hair analysis interpretations that exceed clinical significance, so we recommend staying with a reputable lab. The Prime Level lab kits are excellent. You can order your kit through Better Life Institute (BLI) at www.blionline.com.

2. Order supplements: Make a list of the supplements you need and purchase them online (see appendix D), at a retail outlet, or find a health care practitioner to help you. We enjoyed hearing from one seven-day detoxification enthusiast, Ted Walters, who is the associate director of the BLI. He suggests his clients pick a basic plan of supplements.

Plan A Basic:
A high potency multi vitamin and mineral supplement like:

Double-X	2 sets per day
Milk Thistle	1–2 tabs twice per day

| Antioxidant Complex | 1–2 tabs twice per day |
| Protein Powder | 2–4 scoops (30–60 gms per day) |

For those who want to use a thorough approach and don't mind purchasing a few extra supplements, Ted Walters also suggests a Plan B added to Plan A.

Plan B:

Probiotic Formula	1 packet each meal
Digestive Enzyme	1 with each meal
Omega-3 Fish Oil	2–4 g per day (The recommended FDA dosage for omega-3 is 2 g per day. Doses over 2 g per day need to be on a doctor's recommendation.)
Vitamin C (he recommends the Bio-C Plus)	2–6 tabs per day
CoQ$_{10}$	2–4 tabs per day
Garlic	2–4 tabs per day

After Ted Walter's clients have completed the week of detoxification, he recommends a maintenance plan of:

Double-X	2 sets per day
Milk Thistle	2 tabs per day
Antioxidant Complex	2 tabs per day
Omega-3 Fish Oil	2–4 g per day (see note above regarding omega-3 dosage)

3. Schedule your week of detoxification: Unless you plan your program, it will never happen. The only thing that is important about this program is that you should probably not travel or entertain during this week. Remember to schedule the exercise component into your week. If this is a new addition to your lifestyle, make it easy. Go to a local gym and ask for a qualified person to train you for 3–5 days during this week. Or if you don't feel that you need that type of support, call a friend and ask them to join you for a walk every day at a scheduled time. The help of other people while you are going through a transformative experience is immeasurable.

Obstacles to Your Week of Detoxification

Carrying out the three-module detoxification program isn't easy. You'll need to make some choices that temporarily change how you live. Sticking to a plan requires discipline, and you'll encounter many obstacles, including skepticism and a lack of support from others. The only way to get through these obstacles is by sitting yourself down, reviewing your health problems and your reasons for believing that you might be suffering from toxicity, and then saying to yourself, "I'll do it!"

Choose a week for implementing your plan and make all the necessary arrangements. If necessary, include a friend or spouse in the planning process. Arrange time off from work if you can.

Some of the obstacles that you're likely to encounter include the following:

- Friends and family who might have trouble facing their own lifestyle choices when they see others trying to change their health

- Health care professionals with genuine concern for a patient's welfare who aren't informed about the scientific basis of detoxification therapy and become concerned that this treatment is harmful or a waste of time

- Organizing your daily schedule to a new pattern

- Focusing your willpower to stick with something that's new and causes a little discomfort

The things that you'll miss during your week of detoxification are not important in the context of your whole life. Put into perspective the things that you must give up for that week. The most you'll lose is a few lavish dinners and tasty desserts, but you can have these when the week is done. However, you might be surprised to discover that you don't want them at all. We usually see people making new lifestyle choices after their week on the program, with no desire to go back to their old habits because they feel so good.

The Basic Detoxification Shopping List

In preparation for your EcoTox week, take the following shopping list to the store with you.

- Distilled, filtered, or spring water

- Fresh fruits and vegetables, preferably organic

- Lemons (to make lemon water), preferably organic

- Brown rice (and other "lighter" types of rice, if desired)

- Rice cakes, rice crackers, rice flour bread, rice pasta, rice flour pancake mix

- Herbal teas (nonmedicinal) and green tea

- Bottled organic fruit and vegetable juices

- Rice protein concentrate (sold as a powder)

- Vitamin C, 1,000 mg tablets or capsules

- A multivitamin, containing at least the daily recommended allowance for vitamins A, E, and B-complex and the minerals magnesium, zinc, selenium, and manganese

- Probiotics (*Lactobacillus acidophilus* or *L. bifidus*)

- Milk thistle (200 mg capsules of standardized extract)

- Skin brush

It might be easier to purchase these items through a reputable company like Nutrilite or METAGENICS. One advantage to using Nutrilite products is that they contain many natural ingredients and all of them have phytochemical concentrates, key substances that enhance the detoxification pathways and the utilization of nutrients. You can visit the web site at www.Nutrilite.com or www.Quixtar.com. An independent business owner in your area can make these products available to you by drop shipping them to your door. Nothing could be easier.

Health is not merely the absence of disease. It is a state of optimum organ function that's like money in the bank. Not only do you feel well, but you have a "savings account" to draw on in times of crisis, such as a serious accident or when you come down with an illness. These reserves also help keep you looking and feeling younger. The more you diminish your organ reserves, the faster you will age. By following the seven-day EcoTox plan, you're making a big deposit in your health account. In the next chapter, we'll explain how to modify some of your lifestyle habits so that you can continue to build up your "savings" and increase your organ reserves in the weeks and months following your detoxification program. The choice is up to you.

CHAPTER 9

Recipes and Sample Meal Plan for the Seven-Day Detox Program

One of the main complaints of patients who used the seven-day detox program from the first edition of this book was that there were no recipe guidelines. Putting together a few key ideas about food preparation with recipes was a challenge because we are not the greatest cooks. The ideas presented here may lack depth and originality but are compensated by the fact that they are all easy to prepare and best of all the recipes are *fast!* Many of the basic recipe formulations were created by Cynthia Bennett during her counseling of clinic patients and during the feasts that she would cook for yoga students at weekend classes.

Recipes and Food Ideas

We have eaten all of the wonderful dishes presented in this chapter and can attest to the ease of preparation as well as the excellent taste.

Soups

Bieler Broth

Naturopathic physicians help their patients end an extended fast without experiencing digestive discomfort using this soup.

2 medium zucchini
Handful green beans or spinach
2 stalks celery
1 cup chopped parsley

Steam the zucchini, beans, and celery until soft, about 20 minutes. Place vegetables, steaming water, and parsley into a blender and blend for 1 to 2 minutes until smooth.

Miso Soup

3 cups water
1 carrot
1 onion or leek
1 cup broccoli
Green beans or any other vegetables you like (we often have miso soup with only carrots and onion)
1 cup buckwheat noodles, rice noodles, or bean thread noodles
3 teaspoons miso (use a rice miso)

Boil the water. Add the carrot, onion, broccoli, and any other veggies you have with the noodles. Boil for 10 to 15 minutes. Take off the stove and add the miso. You can use a whisk for this purpose and push it into the miso container. Collect the right amount, then swish it into the soup.

Borscht

>4 cups water
>1 beet
>1 carrot
>1 leek or onion
>½ cup chopped green cabbage
>1 to 2 potatoes
>½ can of tomato paste or canned tomatoes
>Dill weed
>Light miso

Boil the water. Chop the vegetables and add them to the water. Add the tomato paste or canned tomatoes and dill. Cook over medium-low heat until all the vegetables are soft. Just before you are ready to eat, take the soup off the stove and add the miso using the method described in the recipe for miso soup.

Mung Soup

>4 cups water
>1 cup mung beans
>1 onion
>1 carrot
>4 cups water
>Sweet basil
>3 tablespoons miso

Rinse the mung beans. Place the beans along with the other veggies and water in a soup pot. Add the basil and let it go to a boil. After it boils, turn to a lower heat but keep it at a low boil for the next hour. When all veggies are soft, take the pot off the stove and add the miso.

Vegetables and Side Dishes

You can prepare your vegetables by:

Steaming: Place in a pan with ¼ inch of boiling water and cover with a lid for 5 minutes.

Stir Fry: Add 1 tablespoon of olive oil to a hot pan; sauté garlic, onions, and spices; then add the rest of your veggies and ¼ cup of water. Cover with a lid for 5 minutes.

Baking: Place in a Pyrex pan with ¼ inch of water.

Broiling: Place on a cookie sheet, baste a thin coat of olive oil on top of the veggies, and broil for 5 to 10 minutes.

Fresh: Salads, sticks, grated, cubes, mashed, blended.

Coleslaw

> ½ cup cabbage
> ⅛ cup carrots
> ⅛ cup Chinese radish
> ¼ cup cashews
> Vinegar: Enough to make coleslaw wet but not so
>   much that it makes it too sour

Mix the vegetables together. Dry roast the cashews in a toaster oven. When they are cool, add them, with the vinegar, to the cabbage mixture.

Basmati Rice

> *A fragrant South Asian rice.*

> 2 cups water
> 1 cup dry basmati rice

Wash the rice several times in warm water. Put the rice into a pot with water. Heat to the boiling point, then turn to low for the remainder of the cooking time. When the water evaporates, the rice should be done. It takes about 20 minutes.

Gujarati-style Cauliflower

½ cup water
Cauliflower (one serving)
½ teaspoon turmeric
¼ teaspoon mild curry powder
½ teaspoon coriander powder
¼ teaspoon mustard seeds

Cut a serving of cauliflower into small pieces. Dry roast the spices. Place the cauliflower, spices, and water in a pot and cook over medium heat until the cauliflower is done the way you prefer. Some like it overcooked and soft; others like it still a bit crispy.

String Beans with Marinade

½ pound string beans
½ teaspoon lemon juice
1 teaspoon vinegar (brown rice or balsamic)
¼ cup cashews
Flax oil

Cut the beans into 1½-inch pieces. Put into a pot of boiling water and simmer for 10 minutes. Drain the beans and place in a covered baking dish. Combine the other ingredients, except the flax oil, in a small bowl. Pour over the beans and let them sit for 30 minutes, turning the beans so that they are fully covered in sauce. Bake in a 300-degree oven for 30 minutes. Just before serving, pour the flax oil on top.

Salads and Salad Dressings

Mooli Salad

½ cup daikon radish
¼ cup cilantro

On a fine grater, grate enough daikon radish to make ½ cup. Garnish with cilantro.

Oil and Vinegar Dressing

Mix oil and vinegar (8:1) to taste and shake vigorously with dried herbs, such as basil.

Green Dakini Dressing

> ½ cup sunflower seeds, ground
> ½ cup olive oil
> ¼ cup apple cider vinegar
> 2 cups, parsley, chopped
> Garlic powder (optional)
> Salt to taste or 1 tablespoon miso
> Water until desired consistently

Blend all ingredients until smooth. You'll need to add water to thin the mixture. Season to taste. The dressing will thicken if you let it sit for more than 15 minutes. Just add more water if this happens.

Creamy Tofu Dressing

> ½ cube (½ pound) tofu
> ½ cup olive oil
> ¼ cup apple cider vinegar
> Dill weed to taste (this recipe usually requires quite
>   a bit
> ¼ cup poppy seeds
> Garlic powder (optional)
> Salt to taste or 1 tablespoon miso
> Water until desired consistency

Blend all ingredients until smooth. You'll need to add water to thin the mixture. Season to taste. The dressing may thicken if you leave it sitting too long. Just add more water if this happens.

Creamy Dill Dressing

½ cup sunflower seeds, ground
½ cup olive oil
¼ cup apple cider vinegar
½ cup dill weed
2 tablespoons garlic powder
1 tablespoon miso
Water until desired consistently

Blend all ingredients until smooth. You'll need to add water to thin the mixture. Season to taste. The dressing will thicken if it sits for too long. Just add more water if this happens.

Gravy and Sauce

Rice Gravy

¼ cup rice flour
1 cup water
½ teaspoon cumin
½ teaspoon turmeric
4 tablespoons flax oil (or olive oil)
Salt to taste

In a cast-iron frying pan, dry roast the flour until it takes on a light brown color and smells lightly roasted. Take the roasted flour and mix in blender with the water and spices. Then empty into a saucepan and cook over medium heat until the mixture thickens. Cook for another 10 minutes over medium-low heat. Take the gravy off the stove and when cool add the flax or olive oil. Add salt and enjoy!

Tahini Sauce

> 2 to 3 cloves garlic
> ¼ cup tahini
> 4 tablespoons lemon juice
> 4 tablespoons water
> 1 tablespoon finely chopped parsley

Crush the garlic with a press or mince, then crush with a knife blade. Mix all ingredients together. They should form a creamy mixture, the consistency of very heavy cream.

Main Dishes

Pancakes

> *Easy, quick, and very filling.*

> 2 cups buckwheat flour
> 1 teaspoon arrowroot powder (binds and thickens)
> 2 teaspoon baking powder
> 1 tablespoon oil
> 1½ cups water

Mix all ingredients to form a thin batter. Laddle the batter on to a medium-hot grill or frying pan. Cook until bubbles stop forming and then flip. The first set of pancakes are ususally "throw aways" because the pan is not the right temperature. Enjoy with brown rice syrup or maple syrup.

Spinach Tofu Quiche

> **Pie Crust**
> 1½ cups pastry flour
> ⅓ cup oil
> ¾ teaspoon salt
> Water until desired consistency

Filling

½ onion chopped
1 pound chopped spinach, frozen or fresh
1 pound tofu
Dill to taste
Water until desired consistency
Pinch of salt
Olive oil?

To make pie crust, mix oil, salt, flour, and a few tablespoons of water and mix to crumbly consistency. Press into pie pan. Now make the pie filling by lightly frying onion in a little olive oil. When transparent, add chopped spinach. When wilted, place in a blender with the tofu and dill. Blend with as much water as it takes to make this mixture the consistency of pudding. Add salt. Pour into unbaked pie shell. Bake for 45 minutes at 350 degrees.

Mung Curry

This is a very tasty dish full of flavor without any of the hot, spicy taste associated with Indian food.

2 cups mung beans
1 teaspoon olive oil
¼ teaspoon cumin
¼ teaspoon turmeric
¼ teaspoon coriander
½ cup water
1 teaspoon grated fresh ginger
1 can tomatoes

Rinse mung beans and cook until soft but still firm. You can add a pinch of baking soda to the cooking water so that they will cook more quickly. Heat olive oil and spices in a skillet. The mixture will soon smoke and steam. Add water and cover for 15 to 20 minutes. Check that it does not burn. Add ginger and tomatoes. Add beans, drained of their cooking water. Cook over a low heat for at least ½ hour.

Baked Falafel

> 2 cups garbanzo beans
> Juice of 1 lemon
> 1 clove of garlic
> 1 teaspoon coriander
> 1 teaspoon cumin
> ¼ cup of minced celery
> ¼ cup of onion

Take 2 cups cooked garbanzo beans and put them into a food processor or blender or smash them up with a fork. Add juice of lemon and clove of garlic. Add coriander and cumin. After the mixture is smooth, add ¼ cup each minced celery and onion. If the mixture is too loose, add some rice flour. The consistency should be that of stiff dough. Roll into 1-inch-diameter balls and then smash flat with a fork on a cookie sheet. Bake at 400 degrees for 20 minutes or until they look brown around the edges.

Rice Sesame Casserole

> ½ cup of cashews
> Water until desired consistency
> 1 teaspoon dill weed
> 1 onion
> ½ pound chopped spinach
> 2 cups cooked brown rice
> ¼ cup sesame seeds

Blend the cashews with enough water so that they are thicker than cream but thinner than peanut butter. Add dill. Sauté the onion in water, then add the chopped spinach until it wilts. Mix all the ingredients together except 2 spoonfuls of sesame seeds. Place into a baking dish and sprinkle the remaining seeds on the top. Bake for ½ hour at 350 degrees.

Add any steamed veggie as a side dish, but asparagus would be delicious in spring.

Kasha

A wonderful aromatic dish. This dish is simple but has a lovely taste.

> 1 cup toasted buckwheat groats (if you can't find
>   toasted buckwheat, toast the buckwheat at 250 de-
>   grees for 1 hour)
> 2 cups boiling water

Put the toasted buckwheat groats and 2 cups boiling water in a covered baking dish. Bake in the oven for ½ hour at 350 degrees.

Kitcheree

> 1 cup mung beans
> 1 teaspoon oil
> 1 teaspoon black mustard seeds
> ¼ teaspoon cumin seeds
> ½ teaspoon turmeric
> ½ teaspoon coriander
> ¼ teaspoon whole black pepper
> 4 bay leaves
> Stick of cinnamon
> ½ teaspoon grated fresh ginger
> Pinch of cardamom (2 pods)
> 4 cups boiling water
> 1 cup basmati rice

Wash the beans and rice thoroughly, checking for small rocks. Using as little oil as possible, sauté the black mustard seeds and the cumin seeds until they start to pop. Add the other spices and stir. In a few seconds, the oil will be absorbed. Take off the heat. Add 4 cups of boiling water, then add the beans and cook for 20 minutes, then add the rice. Cook over medium-low heat for 1 hour or until everything is soft and well cooked. If desired, you can add vegetables to this while it is cooking, like potatoes (cubed), tomatoes, carrots, spinach, cilantro, peas, or green beans. The result will look a bit like stiff oatmeal. This is the "chicken soup" of the Indian subcontinent.

Desserts

Smoothies

A fruit smoothie is easy to make and tastes good. It is wonderful to experiment with different recipes that you make up yourself!

1 cup soymilk or nut milk
½ to 1 cup water
½ cup fresh fruit
Rice protein powder

Blend all ingredients in blender on high speed until smooth. Try adding bee pollen, wheat germ, almond or cashew butter, fruit juice, ginseng, barley grass powder—the sky is the limit!

Kheir (Rice Pudding)

Cardamom
Cinnamon stick
Black peppercorns (just a few)
¼ cup raisins
¼ cup cashews
2 cups boiling water
1 cup white basmati rice
2⅛ cups soy milk

Add spices, raisins, and cashews to 2 cups of boiling water, then add the rice. Cook on medium-low heat for 20 minutes. Then add 2 cups soy milk and a sweetener such as rice syrup if desired. Some like their kheir without any sweetener. As the mixture cooks, the rice will fall apart. Make sure the mixture is creamy without being too thick. Add ⅛ cup soy milk to thin out.

Banana Rolls

1 to 2 bananas
½ cup desiccated coconut
½ cup carob powder

Cut 1 or 2 bananas into ⅜-inch slices. Roll the fruit into sifted carob powder and desiccated coconut.

Other dessert ideas:

Frozen desserts: blended frozen bananas with lemon

Fresh Fruit

Agar gels

Sweetener ideas:

Date sugar

Rice syrup

Malt syrup

Maple syrup

Honey

Water strained from soaked raisins

Grated fruit

Snacks

Hummus

This Middle Eastern dish is quick if you use canned garbanzo beans.

1 cup garbanzo beans
⅓ cup sesame butter
2 cloves garlic, chopped
⅓ cup parsley, chopped
Juice of 1 lemon
1 teaspoon cumin
Salt to taste
⅛ teaspoon pepper

Mash beans. Blend in sesame butter. Thin with lemon juice and water until the mixture is the consistency of cooked oatmeal. Use as a vegetable or bread dip or as a sandwich spread.

Rice Cakes and Guacamole

This quick snack satisfies and tastes great!

2 ripe avocados (a little soft if pressed)
Juice of 1 lemon
2 cloves crushed garlic
½ teaspoon salt
½ cup each of chopped tomato, green and red
    pepper, olives, cilantro, and fresh onion
Rice cakes

Peel and mash the avocados. Add the remaining ingredients
and mix well. Spread thickly on the rice cakes.

Other snack ideas:

Fruit

Sunflower seeds and raisins with a glass of water

Almonds and dates with mint tea

Beverages

Almond Milk

*Almond milk is a thin, white nut milk with a delicious mild taste and
can be used in place of milk on cereal or for drinking. Some folks
blanch the almond first to remove the skin; it makes a whiter, creamier
milk. I am too lazy to do that and provide the "quick method" here.*

1 cup raw unsalted almonds
4 cups water

Blend the almonds in about 1 cup of water until smooth.
Gradually add more water and continue blending until all 4
cups of water are added. The less water you use, the thicker it
will be. Strain the blended almond/water mixture through a
fine strainer. Almond milk will keep for three to five days
stored covered in the refrigerator. It can also be frozen and

thawed for later use. Honey may also be added to the mixture to sweeten it slightly.

Fruit Tea

This is a wonderful way to dilute fruit juice and use fresh-tasting zesty herbs in a cold drink.

Red zinger tea bags, hibiscus teabags, or loose herbal
tea blend of your choice
1 quart of fruit juice: orange, peach, grape, apple,
pear, mango, or guava
Water to taste

For a quart-size pitcher, use two tea bags and one container of frozen juice, add water to taste. Use hot or cold water depending on the weather. If you use cold water, let it sit overnight. Keep in fridge.

Other beverage ideas:

Hot Tea

Sparkling water with fresh squeezed lemon, lime, or orange juice

Sparkling water with fruit juice

Fresh squeezed juices made with a juicer

Soy milk

Rice milk

Sample Meal Plan

General meal guidelines:

Breakfast: Pancakes, hot rice cereal, rice puffs with soy milk and fruit, smoothie, or fresh fruit

Lunch: Salad, rice, baked vegetable, soup, and fresh fruit

Dinner: Salad, rice, baked vegetable, soup, and fresh fruit

Seven-Day Meal Plan

The following is a sample meal plan for the seven-day detox program. (Meals for Day 1 and 2 are provided for those who opted not to fast.)

DAY 1

Breakfast: Kheir

Snack: Smoothie or rice protein shake

Lunch: Rice bread and tahini butter, salad, and baked potato

Dinner: Spinach Tofu Quiche, Cole Slaw, herb tea, and Banana Rolls

DAY 2

Breakfast: Pancakes

Snack: Smoothie or rice protein shake

Lunch: Butter lettuce with grated carrots, rice, baked potato and baked apple, fresh fruit

Dinner: Mung Curry, rice, Mooli Salad

DAY 3

Breakfast: Fresh fruit salad with nuts in summer or Kheir in cold seasons

Snack: Smoothie or rice protein shake

Lunch: Mooli Salad, rice, baked beets and potatoes, and fresh fruit

Dinner: Baked falafel and tahini sauce, brown rice, and Miso Soup

DAY 4

Breakfast: Kheir

Snack: Smoothie or rice protein shake

Lunch: Salad, rice, leftover Miso Soup from last night, and fresh fruit

Dinner: Rice Sesame Casserole, steamed vegetables, and green salad

DAY 5

Breakfast: Kheir

Snack: Smoothie or rice protein shake

Lunch: Salad, rice, baked vegetable, soup (choose from recipes listed on pages 240–253), and fresh fruit

Dinner: Borscht, Kasha with Rice Gravy, salad, and steamed vegetables

DAY 6

Breakfast: Leftover Kasha from last night with almonds and soy milk

Snack: Smoothie or rice protein shake

Lunch: Salad, rice, baked sweet potato, leftover Borscht from last night, and fresh fruit

Dinner: Kitcheree, cauliflower, and green salad or Mooli Salad

DAY 7

Breakfast: Kheir

Snack: Smoothie or rice protein shake

Lunch: Salad, rice, baked yam, leftover Kitcheree from last night, and fresh fruit

Dinner: Mung Soup, rice bread, String Beans with Marinade, and green leafy salad with flax oil and lemon juice

CHAPTER 10

Before and After Your Detox Program

- Before: Obstacles to Beginning the Program
- After: I've Done the Program—Now What Do I Do?
- Do I Have to Eat Like This for the Rest of My Life?
- The Importance of Digestion
- What Should I Eat?: Common Questions About Food
- Conclusion

You've invested your time in reading about the seven-day detox program and how it can help you. We hope that we have convinced you it's worth the effort. But if you're like most people you're still hesitant to make the commitment. You may have some additional questions, feel it's too complicated to fit in with your normal routine, envision all sorts of stumbling blocks, and be worried about what happens after the seven-day cleanse. In this chapter, we'll address those concerns, answer the questions our patients typically ask, and offer you some tips for how to manage all the details, before and after your detox program.

Before: Obstacles to Beginning the Program

Distrust in Another "New" Therapy

You might have already seen a variety of doctors and specialists, read many health books, and talked to dozens of friends about your health problems. Each person offered different opinions and advice about healing. You might have taken medications, vitamins, and a variety of cure-alls. Perhaps you've tried acupuncture, Chinese herbs, and homeopathic remedies. If the results have been disappointing, it's easy to feel suspicious of yet another therapy. However, the seven-day EcoTox program—based on the idea that self-healing can happen when you put your normal lifestyle on hold and concentrate all your efforts and energy on internal cleansing—can be more powerful than any other treatment you've tried.

Part of this skepticism lies in the fact that we don't trust the body to heal itself. We don't realize that our aches, pains, and all our other symptoms are telling us that something is wrong. We try to get rid of the symptoms without ever doing anything about the real problem. The EcoTox program uses fasting and rest for every system and organ in the body to treat not only the symptoms but also the root cause of illness. Eliminating junk food, poisons, and irritants to the digestive tract for one week encourages the body to heal itself.

Your body is a silent miracle. Every second it creates millions of new cells. Your liver can pick out a foreign substance from the blood and destroy it in a hundredth of a second! Your body is detoxifying itself right now, but you can neither see it nor feel it. No drug, treatment, doctor, hospital, or clinic can do what the body can do for itself. Every cell, when given the chance, has the potential to self-correct any dysfunction and knows exactly how to do it. Our inborn self-healing mechanisms are the best medicine, and the EcoTox program has been formulated to support that natural capacity.

"I Don't Have the Time"

Our response to people who insist that they don't have the time for the detoxification program is that you must make time for things that are important. Disease doesn't happen all of a sudden. Symptoms accumulate over time, and years of bad habits gradually weaken natural resistance. We tell our patients that they can begin to change their health out-look now. Each of us is responsible for meeting our bodies' physiological needs, needs that go beyond merely lowering cholesterol and doing aerobic exercise. Isn't your health worth a one-week time-out? Wouldn't you give seven days to be symptom free? What would it take to persuade you? In some cases, pain and suffering are the best motivators of all.

Eliminating junk food, poisons, and irritants to the digestive tract for one week encourages the body to heal itself.

One of our patients wanted her husband to come to the clinic for a consultation. He never felt that he could leave work for an appointment. We told her that he had a case of NEP but advised her not to worry. "He'll come in eventually," we said. "We just have to wait for the NEP to pass."

She looked at me with a slightly furrowed brow and asked, "What is NEP?"

"NEP is an abbreviation. It stands for Not Enough Pain."

If you don't think you have time to care for your health using detoxification now, you might be forced to take care of your health later when faced with a serious illness. Your body is like a car: It's possible to drive your car for thousands of miles without changing the oil, but engineers and mechanics will tell you that this is not how the machine was designed to be operated. If you don't maintain the engine, you'll eventually need to buy a new one. A quart of oil is a lot cheaper than a new engine. In the same way, a week of detoxification will cost you much less than the onset of disease.

Many people find that they no longer have strong cravings for many of the foods they gave up during their detox week.

Anyone who has symptoms of poor health but lacks the motivation to do what it takes to get well won't get good results from any system of health care. Healing takes effort, and pain can't be treated until it's acknowledged.

"I Have a Job"

Another common time-related issue is that the pressures and demands of a job leave little or no opportunity for the work of self-healing. Keeping to the program schedule can be difficult for anyone who works, and it poses special challenges to busy entrepreneurs and executives, mothers, and single and working parents. You probably should schedule your week of detoxification well in advance and use the time like you would a vacation.

In fact, try using the EcoTox program for at least one week a year. It might be exactly what you need to keep your mind sharp and your health at its peak—to give you the mental clarity, endurance, and performance ability that you need on the job. On the one hand, you really might not have the time to keep yourself healthy; on the other hand, acute or chronic illness can mean even more hours lost from work no matter what your profession.

It's also possible to keep working while you're doing a seven-day detoxification program if you eat an adequate amount of food (for more on this, see chapter 8).

"It Costs Too Much"

Following the recommendations in this book will cost a modest amount (which will vary from location to location) for supplements and food for your week of detoxification. However, the largest expenditure is not in money but in time. Nonetheless, because the program and its requirements fall outside mainstream medicine, people often view it as an unaffordable or unnecessary extra. However, the decision to spend money on this wellness program is a commitment to your health now and in the future. Is that a waste of money or a frivolous expense?

"They Won't Let Me Do It"

Family members, friends, and physicians who have a genuine concern for your well-being might not agree with your decision to follow a detoxification regimen. Unless they take the time to understand the basis of this treatment or go through it themselves, they will base their criticism and advice on absolutely no experience. If you let them, these well-meaning advisers can undermine your chance to get healthy because they simply don't understand that the Eco-Tox program is a health care strategy that combines common sense with cutting-edge medical research. The low-tech nature of this approach makes it an easy target for legions of cynics and skeptics.

Many patients have failed to complete their treatment program because family members or physicians were not supportive and in some cases even gave suggestions counter to our own. When patients experience a healing reaction, those around them might be even more critical of the program, with the result that the program is discontinued at the most critical point in the process.

For people who face this lack of support, we like to pass on the advice of O. G. Carroll, a renowned naturopathic physician who relied exclusively on detoxification therapies to heal his patients—with remarkable results. On the subject of the detoxification healing crisis, he said, "When the patient comes to this cleansing period called 'reaction,' the best advice I can offer them is to first lock all the doors and unplug the telephone. Second, keep all advisers out. Third, settle down to a total fast for four full days."

It's not easy for people who are not sick or who have conservative medical training to understand or accept healing through detoxification. No precedent for this model of health care exists in American culture, and no scientific framework for it exists in American medicine. In contrast, Germany's government-sponsored health care plan covers the cost of two weeks of detoxification therapy at a hydrotherapy spa each year.

After: I've Done the Program— Now What Do I Do?

Congratulations on completing a program that may change your life. By allowing your blood to be cleaned and filtered through this program, you can be confident that you are caring for your health in the most comprehensive way possible.

After your week of cleansing, life must go on. In this post-detoxification period, it's back to "business as usual." If you have any supplements left over from your weeklong program, finish them up before beginning your "renewed" long-term health program. Now that you have a new focus on your peak potential, it's important to figure out which aspects of this program you can integrate into your daily schedule. It's a good time, with your mind and body clear, to make some decisions and rearrange your priorities for optimum health. It may not be as hard as you imagine to change your eating habits and adopt a healthy lifestyle. This is because when you reset your regulatory mechanisms with detoxification, you no longer need the things that were keeping you going, such as naps and sugary foods for an energy boost. Promise yourself that you'll incorporate the following into your daily routine:

- Twenty minutes of exercise

- Time out for mental relaxation

- Eight 8-oz. glasses of water

- Basic nutritional supplementation: a daily multivitamin, special antioxidant and other nutrients that are specific to your individual needs, and an extra 1,000 mg of vitamin C

- Healthy, balanced meals that include adequate protein (60 g), complex carbohydrates (root vegetables and whole grains), and proper fats (omega-3 fatty acids from flax and fish)

Do I Have to Eat Like This for the Rest of My Life?

You may be surprised to discover how well you've adapted to the EcoTox diet. Many people find that they no longer have strong cravings for many of the foods they gave up during their detox week. But changing what you eat and when you eat can be difficult because it affects everyone around you. This may be the biggest hurdle you'll face in living your new, more healthful life. Much of our social interaction takes place around eating. Certain foods are part of every get-together, and we associate them with good times.

Our advice is to do the best you can. Make some guidelines for yourself, follow them when you can and as often as you can, be flexible when necessary, and don't worry about every bite. Some very ill patients must disregard social conventions and follow strict recommendations that don't allow them to adapt to the eating habits of others. People who are highly allergic to certain foods shouldn't eat them—ever. But for the rest of us, eating foods that provide for all of the body's nutritional and digestive requirements is an option: The more often we choose it, the better we feel. Eating the right diet is the first step, but digesting it properly is critical for your long-term health.

The Importance of Digestion

Digestion is the remarkable process of extracting necessary nutrients from food and leaving behind the waste. Two common causes of poor digestion are insufficient secretions of hydrochloric acid in the stomach and a sluggish pancreas that does not produce enough digestive enzymes. Any deviation from healthy digestion encourages fermentation and leads to an altered environment in the gut. Localized inflammation can result, which impedes the absorption of essential nutrients and allows toxins to inundate the bloodstream.

The process of digestion also affects the body's detoxification capacity in a big way. Poor digestion is probably the main cause for toxicity in the body. Unfortunately, symptoms of poor digestion typically go unnoticed or are not taken seriously. After eating, an uncomfortable sense of fullness, flatulence, abdominal pressure, belching, or a burning sensation in the stomach are all written off with a few antacids. When a meal is followed by a headache, congestion, sleepiness, or mental dullness, we drink a cup of coffee or fall asleep on the couch. We never even consider that there might be a relationship between our depression and the foods we eat. But all these are signs of problems in the gastrointestinal system. If they persist, in time the body's physiology and chemistry are changed. The fermented bacterial poisons of poor digestion have profound effects on the immune system, can bring on disease, and slowly age us.

Signs of improper digestion include:

- Prolapsed abdomen
- Obesity
- Food allergies
- Gallbladder disease
- Persistent fatigue
- Increased intestinal permeability
- Intestinal bacterial overgrowth
- Bowel diseases
- Constipation

- Headaches
- Allergies
- Anemia
- Cancer
- Colic
- Immune disorders
- Liver disorders
- Accelerated aging

Digestive Support

As discussed in chapters 7 and 8, it's important to methodically identify foods that do not digest well. After seven days of detoxification, you can eliminate them from your diet permanently.

Because digestion plays such a vital role in our health, meals should be prepared with the same care a pharmacist uses to prepare medicine. The foods you select as well as the way in which they are cooked, served, and eaten influence the effectiveness of digestion.

Visual Appearance   Digestion starts in the eyes. How food looks is important because the sight of it stimulates the brain to begin secreting digestive enzymes.

Smell   The good smells that accompany good-tasting food prompt the salivary glands in the mouth to get busy. Saliva softens food and starts the process of breaking down starches. A side benefit of improved health is a better sense of smell.

Taste   Like visual appeal and smell, taste is extremely important in determining how well foods will digest. People who are very toxic are less sensitive to taste and often choose those that will be hard for them to digest. Healthy people tend to enjoy the taste of healthy foods.

Chewing   Food that isn't chewed thoroughly doesn't get coated with saliva, which contains enzymes needed for proper digestion. In addition, saliva contains a substance called epidermal growth factor (EGF). It is produced only in the salivary glands and is a potent stimulator of cell growth in the liver. Chewing food completely will encourage EGF production. There are many documented cases of seriously ill patients who have shown dramatic improvement as a result of consistently chewing their food well.

Temperature   Excessively cold foods impede blood circulation in the stomach and intestines; avoid them. Foods taken from the refrigerator should be allowed to reach room temperature before being eaten. Drinks should never be taken with ice, especially when they accompany a meal.

   The appetites of children who are fussy eaters will sometimes improve if their parents stop giving them so many cold foods.

Posture   Sitting erect aids digestion by taking pressure off the abdomen and allowing food and air to move freely. Poor digestion affects posture. We adapt to the discomfort of intestinal distress by shifting our weight and altering how we carry ourselves. Often posture improves following detoxification.

Overeating   Eating the right amount of food is just as important as eating the right type of food, and most people consume more than they need. Before real hunger pangs signal that the last meal has been digested, we snack or eat another meal. Our digestive systems never get a rest. Two main meals per day and two snacks are adequate for most adults unless they're doing intense physical training. Studies have shown that reducing our food intake by 30 percent without compromising on essential nutrients such as vitamins, minerals, and antioxidants will increase our life span by 50 percent. If you know you're going out for dinner, for example, skip lunch and instead have only a little snack. You'll arrive at the dinner table with a strong appetite, ready to digest the evening's food properly. In India there's a saying: "Those who can digest it can't afford it, and those who can afford it can't digest it!" Eat at regular intervals, but skip a meal if you aren't hungry.

A pattern of overeating often begins in childhood. Sadness, loneliness, and unhappiness can prompt habitual overeating. People become dependent on this type of neurotic eating as a way to comfort themselves. If you choose the right type of food, eat slowly, and chew completely, you are more likely to eat the right amount of food. Always leave a little room in the stomach. Experiment by eating slightly less than you normally do at each meal. Wait twenty minutes. If you're still hungry, you can eat more, but you may find that you're quite satisfied.

Setting and Atmosphere   Tension and agitation disturb digestion. Upsetting subjects and distressing feelings should not be discussed at mealtimes. Eating while working, watching television, or driving guarantees that food won't be properly digested.

Eat Early, Not Late   Eating a large meal at night makes it impossible to sleep properly and causes indigestion and the fermentation of food in the gut. It keeps the digestive system working all night, which prevents the liver from cleaning the blood of toxins. When you awaken the next day, you feel tired and hung over. It's best to eat the heaviest meal of the day in the afternoon. If that's not possible, be sure to have dinner in the early part of the evening, and don't eat again before going to bed. Eating before going to sleep also causes weight gain. If you must eat in the latter part of the evening, go for a walk after the meal: It helps stimulate the digestive process, especially if you've overeaten.

Cooking The preferable methods of cooking are steaming, poaching, baking, and stir-frying (a technique of quick frying foods over high heat using a small amount of oil followed by the addition of water or broth to complete the cooking process by steaming). Avoid broiling, cooking over charcoal, and deep-frying. We suggest exploring the cuisines of China and Japan for information about healthful cooking methods.

Eating Guidelines The following suggestions will make eating more pleasant and healthful:

- Make food beautiful to the eye and pleasing to the nose

- Eat only when hungry

- Stop eating before you feel stuffed

- Allow at least half an hour to eat

- Take small bites and chew well

- Avoid being distracted while eating

- Sit up straight when eating

- When eating with others, keep the atmosphere relaxed and positive

- Don't eat late at night

- Don't eat very cold foods

- Choose fresh, nutritious foods

- Use healthful cooking methods

What Should I Eat?: Common Questions About Food

After you finish the EcoTox program, your body will tell you what to eat and what to avoid. You'll find yourself instinctually craving foods that are good for you. When you eat a food that's not suited to your constitution, digestive discomfort or other symptoms will arise immediately. If you are healthy, eat a diet that is based on common sense. Avoid sugars, use the right type of fats, get enough protein, eat fresh foods, and enjoy your meals. In our clinic, we recommend a post-detoxification diet rich in fresh vegetables, unrefined grains, nuts, legumes, moderate amounts of fresh fruit; adequate protein from eggs, fish, chicken, and red meat in moderate quantities; and small amounts of healthy fats such as olive oil, nut oils, grape seed oil, and sunflower seed oil. We strongly urge people to eliminate or drink very little alcohol, caffeinated beverages, and soda.

- *Should I eat dairy products?*

Many people eat dairy products and feel healthy. However, we have found that intolerance of cow's milk and products made from it is very widespread, and so we generally do not recommend them to any of our patients. We have noticed, however, that some dairy products, such as Parmesan and mozzarella cheese, are well tolerated, and often those who are sensitive to cow's milk can use goat's milk and cheeses made from it without any problem.

The best way to determine if you should be eating dairy foods is to avoid them completely for one month. If you feel generally better or notice the disappearance of any chronic symptoms such as nasal or chest congestion, skin rashes, or aching joints, they are probably not good for you. To be sure, slowly add them to your diet again and see if you notice any recurrence of symptoms.

- *Are meat, poultry, and fish unhealthy foods? I'm not a vegetarian and don't want to become one.*

We have many vegetarian patients who are surprised when we recommend that they begin eating a meat diet. Poultry, red meat, and fish are excellent forms of nutrition for some individuals, especially if they've been sick. Although personally and philosophically we do not believe in killing animals, it is a clinical fact that some people must eat animal protein to regain and maintain their health. Whenever possible, select meat and poultry from animals that have been grain-fed and are drug-free. If you're a heavy meat eater, try cutting back and balancing your diet with other foods.

Poor digestion is probably the main cause for toxicity in the body.

- *I've heard that proteins and carbohydrates shouldn't be eaten in the same meal. Is it important?*

This idea, which has recently gained some popularity, misses the point: Eat what you can digest. Simple meals are the easiest to digest. When proteins and carbohydrates are eaten together, it makes a big demand on the digestive system and may impede the breakdown of protein. Separating proteins and carbohydrates helps some people. It's recommended only as a possible solution for those with chronic digestive distress.

- *How much sugar is safe to eat?*

Theoretically, no amount of refined sugar, however small, is good for your health. Sugar consumption, along with other refined carbohydrates and artificial sweeteners, is a risk factor for every disease and contributes to obesity. Sugar also ages us through a biochemical phenomenon called glycation reactions. Depending on your genetics, you might be highly susceptible to wide fluctuations in your blood sugar and insulin levels, and this can have serious health consequences. Adult-onset diabetes exists in epidemic proportions in North America.

In addition, refined sugar is not a food. Our bodies don't handle it well, and when we eat it instead of real food we nutritionally shortchange ourselves. But in reality, it's extremely difficult to eliminate all sugar from the diet. It's an ingredient in most packaged and processed food products. Sugary foods are part of celebrations and special occasions. It's in our favorite snacks and desserts. And most of us love our sweets. But with willpower, you can gradually cut back on the amount of sugar you consume. Make choices to eat no sugar or less sugar day by day. In time, you may have less of a desire for it.

- *How many calories should I eat if I want to lose weight?*

We don't recommend counting calories, even if you are trying to lose weight. Once you've detoxified your body and tuned your metabolic engines, you'll naturally want to eat the right foods in the quantities that are right for you. This allows your body to naturally "find" its own normal and healthy weight. That weight might not conform to the current standard of anorexically thin perfection, but it will be one that suits you, one that you can maintain comfortably and easily without jeopardizing your well-being. If you eat a healthy diet, you'll never need to diet again. Doesn't that sound appealing?

- *Should I continue taking supplements?*

We recommend that some daily supplementation with essential nutrients is necessary for everyone. Because we are all so different genetically and because we have different occupations and lifestyles, some nutrient needs will vary. For example, many athletes who are internationally ranked have successfully used this detox program. After the seven days, they continue on a supplement program that is very high in essential fatty acids, protein, and minerals. The supplement needs of a competitive athlete are much dfferent than those of a software programmer who sits at a desk all day. For the average person, a multiple vitamin with minerals and antioxidants is sufficient to meet nutritional needs. If you have special health problems that are chronic, you might have to use a supplement program that falls outside the basic needs described previously. For example, patients who are prone to kidney stones find that they are much less prone to the problem if they take extra vitamin B_6 and magnesium on a daily basis. In fact, those who use vitamin B_6 and magnesium sometimes never have another kidney stone for the rest of their life! To provide a long-term nutritional program that will fit the biochemical individuality of all patients is outside the scope of this short chapter and is probably best left to a qualified health professional.

- *Should I continue doing hydrotherapy?*

Our body thrives when there is adequate circulation. Good circulation is the basis of good health. "Stasis is the basis." Whether you attain that good circulation through regular exercise, yoga, sauna baths, or hydrotherapy doesn't matter. More, in this case, is better. The more you stimulate circulation, the healthier you'll be. People who regularly exercise outdoors are healthier, and it shows in the long run, as they age with few health problems. Each person needs to find the methods that work best for them through trial and error. Who knows, your best form of exercise may be ballroom dancing. You won't know until you try a few different strategies. Whatever you do, it has to be done on a regular basis.

- *Should I continue mind training?*

The power of the mind to heal or harm us is one of the most important factors we need to consider in our overall health. Each person will need to find the method that suits him or her the best. Some people find that going to church and doing daily prayer is what keeps their mind calm and centered. Others relate more to a daily meditation practice like Vipassana meditation. Some need to have a quiet time, a period of reflection to settle their affairs and plunge into their heart to find the center of their self and bask in the inner light they find. Life is short and goes by quickly, so don't wait for a future day to discover and uncover the inner dimension of your being. Make it a priority to include this in your new plans for optimum health.

Conclusion

This book is an operating manual for your body. If you take care of it, according to the instructions and guidelines we've provided, it will give you a lifetime of good health. We have brought together the knowledge of many great doctors, dedicated researchers, and renowned teachers to help you, as well as what we have learned from our many years in practice. We know that the seven-day EcoTox program works. Now is the time for you to find out just what it can do for you. Are you willing to try?

Never before have our bodies been exposed to so many chemicals, pollutants, and drugs. Air, water, soil, and food sources are devitalized and riddled with toxins. Substances generated in the lab and unknown by nature appear on our tables. You've read that the build up of toxins in the body is a health issue for everyone. You now have a strategy for removing them. You know what it will cost, in time, money, and effort, to go through the process of detoxification and how to integrate some of those same cleansing and purifying principles into your daily life. You know why this program has the potential to make you feel much better than you do now, whether you are sick or not. Choosing to read this book is the first step. Following the program is the next. Take that next step. Take charge of your own health by clearing your body of toxins and nourish every system, organ, and cell, and a week later, we're certain that you'll agree that this is truly a seven-day miracle.

APPENDIX A:
DETOXIFICATION
QUESTIONNAIRE

Totals

1. How often are you exposed to petrochemicals? ____
   a) Rarely   b) Weekly   c) Daily

2. How often are you exposed to pesticides? ____
   a) Rarely   b) Weekly   c) Daily

3. How often are you exposed to air pollution? ____
   a) Rarely   b) Weekly   c) Daily

4. How much time do you spend in cities? ____
   a) 1–2 days a month
   b) 1–3 days a week
   c) 4–7 days a week

5. How often do you take prescription medication
   or over-the-counter medication? ____
   a) Rarely
   b) Once a month
   c) Once a week or more

6. How often do you skip meals if you are
   not hungry? ____
   a) Never
   b) Once a month
   c) Once a week

7. How often do you eat organic food?   _____
   a) Never (Rarely)
   b) 50 percent of the time
   c) 75 percent of the time or more

8. How often do you eat canned or frozen foods?   _____
   a) Rarely
   b) 5–7 times a month
   c) 3–7 times a week

9. How often do you drink alcohol?   _____
   a) Rarely
   b) Once a week
   c) Once a day or more

10. Do you smoke cigarettes/cigars?   _____
    a) Yes   b) No

11. How often do you exercise?   _____
    a) Less than once a week
    b) 1–2 times a week
    c) 3–5 times a week

12. Do you have mercury amalgam fillings?   _____
    a) Yes   b) No

13. Do you have any root canals?   _____
    a) Yes   b) No

14. Do you suffer from fibromyalgia?   _____
    a) Yes   b) No

15. How often do you suffer from arthritis?   _____
    a) Rarely (Never)   b) Weekly   c) Daily

16. Do you suffer from inflamed bowels?   _____
    a) Yes   b) No

17. How often do you experience indigestion?   _____
    a) Rarely
    b) Once a month
    c) Once a week or more

18. How often do you experience belching/flatulence? _____
    a) Rarely   b) Weekly   c) Daily

19. How often do you experience diarrhea? _____
    a) Rarely   b) Weekly   c) Daily

20. Do you suffer from anemia? _____
    a) Yes   b) No

21. Do you suffer from hepatitis or other
    liver diseases? _____
    a) Yes   b) No

22. Do you suffer from gallbladder disease? _____
    a) Yes   b) No

23. How often do you have dry, tired eyes? _____
    a) Rarely   b) Weekly   c) Daily

24. How often do you have bags under your eyes? _____
    a) Rarely   b) Weekly   c) Daily

25. How often do you have circles under your eyes? _____
    a) Rarely   b) Weekly   c) Daily

26. How often do you have headaches? _____
    a) Rarely   b) Weekly   c) Daily

27. Do you suffer from chemical sensitivities? _____
    a) Yes   b) No

28. Do you suffer from frequent infections? _____
    a) Yes   b) No

29. Do you have chronic fatigue syndrome? _____
    a) Yes   b) No

30. Do you suffer from autoimmune diseases? _____
    a) Yes   b) No

31. Do you have or have you had cancer? _____
    a) Yes   b) No

32. Do you suffer from allergies?   _____
    a) Yes   b) No

33. How often do you suffer from sinus problems?   _____
    a) Rarely   b) Weekly   c) Daily

34. How often do you suffer from a swollen,
    red tongue?   _____
    a) Rarely   b) Weekly   c) Daily

35. How often do you feel apathetic?   _____
    a) Rarely   b) Weekly   c) Daily

36. How would you rate your energy level?   _____
    a) High   b) Moderate   c) Low

37. How would you rate your mental acuity?   _____
    a) High   b) Moderate   c) Low

38. How often do you notice that you have
    poor concentration?   _____
    a) Rarely   b) Weekly   c) Daily

39. Do you have a poor memory?   _____
    a) Yes   b) No

40. How often do you suffer from drowsiness?   _____
    a) Rarely   b) Weekly   c) Daily

41. How often do you get angry or irritable?   _____
    a) Rarely   b) Weekly   c) Daily

42. How often do you have mood swings?   _____
    a) Rarely   b) Weekly   c) Daily

43. How often do you feel depressed?   _____
    a) Rarely   b) Weekly   c) Daily

44. How often do you suffer from insomnia?   _____
    a) Rarely   b) Weekly   c) Daily

45. How often do you feel groggy upon waking? _____
    a) Rarely   b) Weekly   c) Daily

46. How often do you feel that it is difficult to relax? _____
    a) Rarely   b) Weekly   c) Daily

47. How often do you suffer from excessive stress? _____
    a) Rarely   b) Weekly   c) Daily

Scoring Key:

1. a=0 b=5 c=10	17. a=0 b=1 c=2	33. a=0 b=2 c=4
2. a=0 b=5 c=10	18. a=0 b=1 c=2	34. a=0 b=1 c=2
3. a=0 b=2 c=4	19. a=0 b=2 c=5	35. a=0 b=1 c=2
4. a=0 b=1 c=2	20. a=3 b=0	36. a=0 b=2 c=5
5. a=0 b=2 c=4	21. a=10 b=0	37. a=0 b=2 c=5
6. a=2 b=1 c=-2	22. a=2 b=0	38. a=0 b=2 c=5
7. a=3 b=1 c=-5	23. a=0 b=1 c=2	39. a=5 b=0
8. a=0 b=1 c=2	24. a=0 b=1 c=2	40. a=0 b=1 c=2
9. a=0 b=1 c=2	25. a=0 b=1 c=2	41. a=0 b=1 c=2
10. a=2 b=0	26. a=0 b=1 c=2	42. a=0 b=2 c=5
11. a-2 b=1 c=-3	27. a=5 b=0	43. a=0 b=2 c=5
12. a=4 b=0	28. a=5 b=0	44. a=0 b=1 c=2
13. a=3 b=0	29. a=7 b=0	45. a=0 b=2 c=5
14. a=5 b=0	30. a=10 b=0	46. a=0 b=1 c=2
15. a=0 b=2 c=4	31. a=10 b=0	47. a=0 b=3 c=5
16. a=2 b=0	32. a=3 b=0	

Score of 101 or more: Your lifestyle predisposes you to toxic buildup in your system. You are also showing elevated symptoms and risk factors for toxic accumulation. It is recommended that you reassess your lifestyle and implement the EcoTox program into your schedule every three months.

Score of 66–100: Although you are not in as toxic a state as you would be if you were to score more than 100, you still have a lifestyle that predisposes you to toxicity and are already showing symptoms and risk factors for toxic accumulation. It is recommended that you reassess your lifestyle and implement the EcoTox program into your schedule every four months.

Score of 31–65: Your score on this questionnaire shows that you are a generally healthy person. However, you are either showing some symptoms or have a lifestyle that predisposes you to toxicity. It is recommended that you assess your life for any possible changes that could be made and follow the EcoTox program every six months.

Score of 30 or less: Congratulations, you are living in a way that is very beneficial to your health. As a result, you are not showing any symptoms of toxicity. To continue this preventive lifestyle it is recommended that you follow the EcoTox program once a year.

*Note: This questionnaire is not a replacement for primary care medical screening.

APPENDIX B:
IMPLEMENTING A
DETOXIFICATION PROGRAM

The two main requests from patients and long-distance readers who sent in their feedback of the first edition of this book was for the addition of recipes and for a checklist program, something that you could tape to your fridge and follow during the week without having to do too much thinking. There is so much information in the book and, without this tool, some people had a nagging anxiety that they were missing something or had forgotten some part of the program. It is a sort of "plug and play" version of good health.

Sample Seven-Day schedule
for the EcoTox Program

This is a sample daily schedule assuming that you get 9 hours of sleep, work 8 hours, and have minimal responsibility (extracurricular activity, entertaining, child rearing).

Days 1 and 2

Time	Liquid
7 A.M.	8 oz. Lemon water
8 A.M.	
9 A.M.	8 oz. Lemon water
10 A.M.	
11 A.M.	8 oz. Lemon water
12 P.M.	
1 P.M.	8 oz. Lemon water
2 P.M.	
3 P.M.	8 oz. Lemon water
4 P.M.	
5 P.M.	8 oz. Lemon water
6 P.M.	
7 P.M.	8 oz. Lemon water
8 P.M.	
9 P.M.	8 oz. Lemon water
10 P.M.	

Time	Food
7 A.M.	None for the day
8 A.M.	
9 A.M.	
10 A.M.	
11 A.M.	
12 P.M.	
1 P.M.	
2 P.M.	
3 P.M.	

4 P.M.

5 P.M.

6 P.M.

7 P.M.

8 P.M.

9 P.M.

10 P.M.

Time	Activity
7 A.M.	Wake up, shower/hydrotherapy/mind training
8 A.M.	Short 20-minute walk
9 A.M.	Read/rest
10 A.M.	Read/rest
11 A.M.	Read/rest
12 P.M.	Short 20-minute walk
1 P.M.	Read/rest
2 P.M.	Read/rest
3 P.M.	Read/rest
4 P.M.	Read/rest
5 P.M.	Shower/hydrotherapy
6 P.M.	Read/rest
7 P.M.	20-minute walk
8 P.M.	Read/rest
9 P.M.	Read/rest
10 P.M.	Hydrotherapy/bedtime

Day 3

Time	Liquid
7 A.M.	8 oz. Lemon water
8 A.M.	
9 A.M.	8 oz. Lemon water
10 A.M.	
11 A.M.	8 oz. Lemon water
12 P.M.	
1 P.M.	8 oz. Lemon water
2 P.M.	
3 P.M.	8 oz. Lemon water
4 P.M.	
5 P.M.	8 oz. Lemon water
6 P.M.	
7 P.M.	
8 P.M.	8 oz. Lemon water
9 P.M.	
10 P.M.	

Time	Food
7 A.M.	
8 A.M.	Breakfast: Kheir and fruit
9 A.M.	
10 A.M.	Snack: Rice protein shake
11 A.M.	
12 P.M.	Lunch: Rice bread and tahini butter, salad, baked potato
1 P.M.	

2 P.M.	
3 P.M.	Snack: Rice protein shake
4 P.M.	
5 P.M.	
6 P.M.	Dinner: Spinach tofu quiche, coleslaw, herb tea, banana rolls
7 P.M.	
8 P.M.	
9 P.M.	
10 P.M.	

Time	Activity
7 A.M.	Wake/shower/hydrotherapy/mind training
8 A.M.	
9 A.M.	
10 A.M.	
11 A.M.	
12 P.M.	
1 P.M.	
2 P.M.	
3 P.M.	
4 P.M.	
5 P.M.	Exercise/hydrotherapy
6 P.M.	
7 P.M.	
8 P.M.	
9 P.M.	
10 P.M.	

Time	Supplements
7 A.M.	
8 A.M.	Multivitamin, milk thistle, antioxidant, acidophilus
9 A.M.	
10 A.M.	
11 A.M.	
12 P.M.	Multivitamin, milk thistle, antioxidant, acidophilus
1 P.M.	
2 P.M.	
3 P.M.	
4 P.M.	
5 P.M.	
6 P.M.	Multivitamin, milk thistle, antioxidant, acidophilus
7 P.M.	
8 P.M.	
9 P.M.	
10 P.M.	

Day 4

Time	Liquid
7 A.M.	8 oz. Lemon water
8 A.M.	
9 A.M.	8 oz. Lemon water
10 A.M.	
11 A.M.	8 oz. Lemon water
12 P.M.	

1 P.M.	8 oz. Lemon water
2 P.M.	
3 P.M.	8 oz. Lemon water
4 P.M.	
5 P.M.	8 oz. Lemon water
6 P.M.	
7 P.M.	
8 P.M.	8 oz. Lemon water
9 P.M.	
10 P.M.	

Time	Food
7 A.M.	
8 A.M.	Breakfast: Pancakes
9 A.M.	
10 A.M.	Snack: Rice protein shake
11 A.M.	
12 P.M.	Lunch: Butter lettuce with grated carrots, rice, baked potato and baked apple, fresh fruit
1 P.M.	
2 P.M.	
3 P.M.	Snack: Rice protein shake
4 P.M.	
5 P.M.	
6 P.M.	Dinner: Mung curry, rice, mooli salad
7 P.M.	
8 P.M.	
9 P.M.	
10 P.M.	

Time	Activity
7 A.M.	Wake up/shower/hydrotherapy/mind training
8 A.M.	
9 A.M.	
10 A.M.	
11 A.M.	
12 P.M.	
1 P.M.	
2 P.M.	
3 P.M.	
4 P.M.	
5 P.M.	Exercise/hydrotherapy
6 P.M.	
7 P.M.	
8 P.M.	
9 P.M.	
10 P.M.	

Time	Supplements
7 A.M.	
8 A.M.	Multivitamin, milk thistle, antioxidant, acidophilus
9 A.M.	
10 A.M.	
11 A.M.	
12 P.M.	Multivitamin, milk thistle, antioxidant, acidophilus
1 P.M.	

2 P.M.	
3 P.M.	
4 P.M.	
5 P.M.	
6 P.M.	Multivitamin, milk thistle, antioxidant, acidophilus
7 P.M.	
8 P.M.	
9 P.M.	
10 P.M.	

Day 5

Time	Liquid
7 A.M.	8 oz. Lemon water
8 A.M.	
9 A.M.	8 oz. Lemon water
10 A.M.	
11 A.M.	8 oz. Lemon water
12 P.M.	
1 P.M.	8 oz. Lemon water
2 P.M.	
3 P.M.	8 oz. Lemon water
4 P.M.	
5 P.M.	8 oz. Lemon water
6 P.M.	
7 P.M.	
8 P.M.	8 oz. Lemon water
9 P.M.	
10 P.M.	

Time	Food
7 A.M.	
8 A.M.	Breakfast: Kheir
9 A.M.	
10 A.M.	Snack: Rice protein shake
11 A.M.	
12 P.M.	Lunch: Salad, rice, baked vegetable, soup, fresh fruit
1 P.M.	
2 P.M.	
3 P.M.	Snack: Rice protein shake
4 P.M.	
5 P.M.	
6 P.M.	Dinner: Borscht, kasha with rice gravy, salad, steamed vegetables
7 P.M.	
8 P.M.	
9 P.M.	
10 P.M.	

Time	Activity
7 A.M.	Wake up/shower/hydrotherapy/mind training
8 A.M.	
9 A.M.	
10 A.M.	
11 A.M.	
12 P.M.	
1 P.M.	
2 P.M.	

3 P.M.

4 P.M.

5 P.M.   Exercise/hydrotherapy

6 P.M.

7 P.M.

8 P.M.

9 P.M.

10 P.M.

Time	Supplements
7 A.M.	
8 A.M.	Multivitamin, milk thistle, antioxidant, acidophilus
9 A.M.	
10 A.M.	
11 A.M.	
12 P.M.	Multivitamin, milk thistle, antioxidant, acidophilus
1 P.M.	
2 P.M.	
3 P.M.	
4 P.M.	
5 P.M.	
6 P.M.	Multivitamin, milk thistle, antioxidant, acidophilus
7 P.M.	
8 P.M.	
9 P.M.	
10 P.M.	

Day 6

Time	Liquid
7 A.M.	8 oz. Lemon water
8 A.M.	
9 A.M.	8 oz. Lemon water
10 A.M.	
11 A.M.	8 oz. Lemon water
12 P.M.	
1 P.M.	8 oz. Lemon water
2 P.M.	
3 P.M.	8 oz. Lemon water
4 P.M.	
5 P.M.	8 oz. Lemon water
6 P.M.	
7 P.M.	
8 P.M.	8 oz. Lemon water
9 P.M.	
10 P.M.	

Time	Food
7 A.M.	
8 A.M.	Breakfast: Kasha from last night with almonds and soy milk
9 A.M.	
10 A.M.	Snack: Rice protein shake
11 A.M.	
12 P.M.	Lunch: Salad, rice, baked sweet potato, borscht from last night, fresh fruit

1 P.M.	
2 P.M.	
3 P.M.	Snack: Rice protein shake
4 P.M.	
5 P.M.	
6 P.M.	Dinner: Kitcheree, cauliflower, green salad or mooli salad
7 P.M.	
8 P.M.	
9 P.M.	
10 P.M.	

Time	Activity
7 A.M.	Wake up/shower/hydrotherapy/mind training
8 A.M.	
9 A.M.	
10 A.M.	
11 A.M.	
12 P.M.	
1 P.M.	
2 P.M.	
3 P.M.	
4 P.M.	
5 P.M.	Exercise/hydrotherapy
6 P.M.	
7 P.M.	
8 P.M.	
9 P.M.	
10 P.M.	

Time	Supplements
7 A.M.	
8 A.M.	Multivitamin, milk thistle, antioxidant, acidophilus
9 A.M.	
10 A.M.	
11 A.M.	
12 P.M.	Multivitamin, milk thistle, antioxidant, acidophilus
1 P.M.	
2 P.M.	
3 P.M.	
4 P.M.	
5 P.M.	
6 P.M.	Multivitamin, milk thistle, antioxidant, acidophilus
7 P.M.	
8 P.M.	
9 P.M.	
10 P.M.	

Day 7

Time	Liquid
7 A.M.	8 oz. Lemon water
8 A.M.	
9 A.M.	8 oz. Lemon water
10 A.M.	
11 A.M.	8 oz. Lemon water

12 P.M.	
1 P.M.	8 oz. Lemon water
2 P.M.	
3 P.M.	8 oz. Lemon water
4 P.M.	
5 P.M.	8 oz. Lemon water
6 P.M.	
7 P.M.	
8 P.M.	8 oz. Lemon water
9 P.M.	
10 P.M.	

Time	Food
7 A.M.	
8 A.M.	Breakfast: Kheir
9 A.M.	
10 A.M.	Snack: Rice protein shake
11 A.M.	
12 P.M.	Lunch: Salad, rice, baked yams, kitcheree from last night, fresh fruit
1 P.M.	
2 P.M.	
3 P.M.	Snack: Rice protein shake
4 P.M.	
5 P.M.	
6 P.M.	Dinner: Mung soup, rice bread, string beans with marinade, green leafy salad with flax oil and lemon juice
7 P.M.	

8 P.M.

9 P.M.

10 P.M.

Time	Activity
7 A.M.	Wake up/shower/hydrotherapy/mind training
8 A.M.	
9 A.M.	
10 A.M.	
11 A.M.	
12 P.M.	
1 P.M.	
2 P.M.	
3 P.M.	
4 P.M.	
5 P.M.	Exercise/hydrotherapy
6 P.M.	
7 P.M.	
8 P.M.	
9 P.M.	
10 P.M.	

Time	Supplements
7 A.M.	
8 A.M.	Multivitamin, milk thistle, antioxidant, acidophilus
9 A.M.	

10 A.M.	
11 A.M.	
12 P.M.	Multivitamin, milk thistle, antioxidant, acidophilus
1 P.M.	
2 P.M.	
3 P.M.	
4 P.M.	
5 P.M.	
6 P.M.	Multivitamin, milk thistle, antioxidant, acidophilus
7 P.M.	
8 P.M.	
9 P.M.	
10 P.M.	

A Journal of One Woman's Experience on the EcoTox Program

The following is a journal kept by Jacqueline Allan of British Columbia during her seven-day detoxification program. Each individual's experiences will be different, but this may give you some idea of what to expect.

JANUARY 12, 2001: PREVIEW DAY
No illness, good energy, sleeping well, 135 lbs. Ate only raw foods and distilled water with lemon to prepare for two-day fast. 10km walk and sauna.

JANUARY 13: DAY ONE

Fasting—felt calmer and physically more relaxed than is usual for me. Had two short naps to keep me charged, in bed at 8:30 P.M. Slept deeply, peacefully, until a most uncharacteristic 9 A.M. Sense of smell was heightened all through this first day, the world seemed to slow down around me. No strong desire to eat. Attended a birthday celebration with lavish foods and cake and did not find it difficult to continue plan amidst all this.

JANUARY 14: DAY TWO

Slept until 8:30 A.M. (4 hours longer than my typical 4:30 A.M. start. My body feels happy and at peace, my pace is slow today, but I am keeping up with my responsibilities. Made breakfast, lunch, and dinner for my family and joined them comfortably at the table. Did have to pace myself, but no headache, no body aches, no abdominal distress whatsoever. Tummy is quiet and undisturbed.

My extremities are cold, a heating bath was necessary to stay comfortable, the ten-minute warm soak was energizing. I highly recommend it (particularly during the fasting). Asleep by 8:30 P.M. (this is usual). Feel great.

JANUARY 15: DAY THREE

Awake at 4:00 A.M. Feel fresh and rested, walked 10 km, mind/breath training, dry brush, lemon water as per usual. The two-day break from food has me keen to continue fasting, will adhere to program and break my fast today. No desire to eat, no aches or troubles. My energy remains more even throughout the day.

JANUARY 16: DAY FOUR

Feel terrific! Did three-hour yoga practice, eating fresh fruit, lots of steamed greens, kale, Swiss chard, collard greens with baked beets, yams, artichokes, salads. Have had very little juice other than prescribed lemon water.

JANUARY 17: DAY FIVE

I'm sleeping longer (this is different), but I am accommodating this need just now. Common to all five days thus far is a noticeable ease systemically and emotionally. My strong tenacious drive has been softened. I feel different, nicely so.

JANUARY 18: DAY SIX

Awoke feeling that my body was out of balance and struggling, feet and hands slightly puffy. Vague (mild) unwell feeling. Walked long and fast in the fresh air, long sauna, lemon water, cold shower, more sauna, and a short rest— this seemed to rectify how I was feeling. Stayed on track with program requirements, appetite disappeared today. Comments from others that I'm looking tired validated my need to rest more today, retired early. Bowels moving comfortably and regularly, my sleep seems especially deep and peaceful.

JANUARY 19: DAY SEVEN

This seventh day came surprisingly quick and with no desire to discontinue the routine established over the week. Although each individual's experience will be their own, this was not about hardships for me. I feel that I've tasted the potential for consistent, even energy throughout the day. It is exciting to know there is still more I can do to achieve higher levels of energy and wellness. Was genuinely surprised by how I felt right through each day until bedtime. Activity wise—I said yes to more each day. General ease in my body and mind. Very satisfied to have had this experience and expect to integrate much of what is prescribed in the EcoTox program into my life in the days and weeks to come.

This concentrated attention on one's self and diet has freed me from the restraints of low energy and compounding distractions resulting from imbalances, even small ones. 128 lbs. Feel alert and alive!

TESTIMONIAL

What a powerful difference seven days can make! This program has been immediately useful in fine tuning and balancing an already healthy person's body. I am astonished with how much stronger and more healthy I'm feeling. It was not the difficult crucible one might expect in order to achieve such dramatic results. There is a real genius in this seven-day detoxification program. My body's innate ability to repair and "right itself" has been switched on. I can feel it! I learned through the program to fast as if my life depends on it, and now I am so clearly aware that it does. Thank you for how I feel today. Committing myself to continuous improvement, nourishing and maintaining this new-found higher level of health has to be the best way to honor this gift. As terrific as I feel on this seventh day, the program's success is measured in the permanent changes I intend to make in my life as a result of it.

APPENDIX C:
TREATMENT
REPERTOIRE

In this appendix, I have picked several health conditions that respond well to the EcoTox program to give an example of how it might be necessary to adopt an individualized approach to your specific health care concern. For all the health conditions outlined here, use the EcoTox program in combination with the following additions. These recommendations should be used along with the recommendations and supervision of a qualified, licensed health professional and are not meant to suggest that these treatment strategies, as a self-care program, are a replacement for good medical care. Call Dr. Bennett's clinic (250-544-4331) if you have any questions.

Crohn's Disease

Acute cases:

- Rice protein and clear vegetable broth only until bleeding and pain stops

- Herbal demulcents (Robert's Formula 2 caps three times per day)

- Glutamine: 500 mg three times per day

- Pancreatin: one tab with meals

Chronic cases:

- Eliminate food allergies (wheat, dairy, eggs, corn, yeast, brassica vegetables) and candida

- Pancreatin: one tab with meals

- Essential fatty acids (fish oil): 1 g three times per day

- Vitamin E: 800 IU per day

- Glutamine: 500 mg three times per day

- Vitamin B_{12}: 1,000 mg per day

- Vitamin A: 30,000 IU per day

- Folic acid: 2 to 20 mg per day

- Zinc picolinate: 30 mg twice per day

- Copper: 2 to 4 mg per day

- *Lactobacillus acidophilus/Saccharomyces boulardii:* one dose twice a day

- Multiple vitamin/mineral: once per day

- Curcumin (inhibits lipid peroxidation and increases hepatic glutathione concentrations): 400 mg three times per day

- Green barley powder: 1 teaspoon three times per day in fresh juice

Colitis

Acute cases:

- Rice protein and clear vegetable broth only until bleeding and pain stops

- Herbal demulcents (Robert's Formula: 2 caps three times per day)

- Glutamine: 500 mg three times per day

- Vitamin A: 100,000 IU per day for 3 weeks and then taper down to 30,000 IU per day

- Aloe juice: drink three times per day

- Pancreatin: one tab with meals

Chronic cases:

- Eliminate food allergies (wheat, dairy, eggs, corn, yeast, brassica vegetables) and candida

- Pancreatin: one tab with meals

- Essential fatty acids (fish oil): 1 g three times per day

- Vitamin E: 800 IU per day

- Glutamine: 500 mg three times per day

- Vitamin B_{12}: 1,000 mg per day

- Vitamin A: 30,000 IU per day

- Folic acid: 2 to 20 mg per day

- Zinc picolinate: 30 mg twice per day

- Copper: 2 to 4 mg per day

- *Lactobacillus acidophilus/Saccharomyces boulardii*

- Multiple vitamin/mineral

- Curcumin (inhibits lipid peroxidation and increases hepatic glutathione concentrations): 400 mg three times per day

- Green barley powder: 1 teaspoon three times per day in fresh juice

Fatigue

Get a good diagnosis. The following are the main causes of fatigue seen in my clinic:

- Epstein-Barr virus

- CMV (cytomegalovirus)

- Candida

- Chronic disease

- Depression

- High or low blood sugar or high insulin

- Vitamin and mineral deficiency

- Food allergies

- Adrenal and DHEA insufficiencies

- Dysbiosis

- Hypothyroidism

- Protein deficiency

- Anemia

If all these are ruled out, use the seven-day detoxification program, making sure to use adequate rice protein shakes during the seven days. Add the following:

- Vitamin B_{12} injections three times per week for one month

- Strict avoidance of sugar, caffeine, alcohol, and refined foods (white flour) for three months

- DHEA if levels are low

- Potassium and magnesium aspartate: 100 mg each twice per day

Fibromyalgia

Fibromyalgia simply means that your muscles hurt for some unknown reason. It is defined as nonarticular rheumatism characterized by widespread musculoskeletal aching and stiffness as well as tenderness on pressure at tender points. Fibromyalgia is usually diagnosed when the pains are of greater than three months' duration, usually accompanied by fatigue and anxiety or depression. There are an estimated three to six million people afflicted with this disorder, the majority of whom are women between 25 and 45 years of age, with females outnumbering males by six to one. These patients tend to present themselves to their physicians as stressed, tense, depressed, and anxious. It may be induced or intensified by physical or mental stress, chronic overwork, poor sleep or sleep disorders, physical or emotional trauma, depression, exposure to dampness or cold, and occasionally by a systemic, usually rheumatic, disorder.

Fibromyalgia is a complex syndrome with no known cause or cure and should probably be called "muscular rheumatism." Any fibromuscular tissues may be involved, but those of the neck, lower back (lumbago), shoulders, thorax (chest pain), and thighs (aches and spasms) are especially affected.

In addition to generalized pain, there is ususaly also stiffness, fatigue, poor sleep, and a sensation of swelling and tingling. Biochemical mechanisms are theorized to be due to increased substance P, decreased serotonin, decreased GABA, decreased norepinephrine, and decreased enkephalins. Some research now indicates that fibromyalgia patients may be deficient in certain nutrients required for the synthesis of adenosine triphosphate (ATP) in the mitochondria. ATP synthesis requires the presence of magnesium, coenzyme Q_{10}, glutathione, and other antioxidants.

Aluminum toxicity may also play a role in symptoms experienced by a magnesium-deficient fibromyalgia patient because magnesium is needed to help the body block the toxic effects of aluminum. Aluminum inhibits glycolysis and oxidative phosphorylation, resulting in decreased intramitochondrial ATP production. Additionally, because of its high affinity for phosphate groups, aluminum blocks the absorption and utilization of phosphates vital to the synthesis of ATP. This further contributes to the problem of intramitochondrial phosphate deficiency.

After completing the detoxification program, you can begin to rule out one or more causes of fibromyalgia:

• Food allergies (wheat, dairy, eggs, corn, yeast)

• Candida

• Toxic metals: mercury is the most common offender in our patients

• Adrenal deficiency leading to severe muscle pain, especially in posttraumatic stress disorder

• Loss of sleep

• Depression

• Vitamin and mineral deficiency

• DHEA insufficiency

• Intestinal microflora imbalance

• Protein deficiency

• Emotional trauma

People suffering from fibromyalgia may find the following supplements helpful:

• Begin a course of magnesium therapy. We have found amazing results from using intravenous magnesium therapy. If possible, have a lab measure magnesium levels using a whole blood elemental analysis.

- Magnesium malate (malic acid is part of the TCA cycle that is needed to increase ATP) with potassium/magnesium aspartate to get rid of lactic acid: 300 mg twice per day.

- Epsom salt baths.

- Selenium: 100 to 250 µ/day with vitamin E.

- Pantothenic acid: 500 mg twice per day.

- Licorice root: ¼ teaspoon per day of solid extract (watch for increased blood pressure).

Chronic and Migraine Headaches

Chronic headaches have several key causes:

1. Musculoskeletal spasm in the neck: Classically starts at the back of the neck and radiates forward with potential secondary vascular spasm.

2. Vascular: Vasoconstriction is commonly caused by coffee, alcohol, chocolate, wine, and beer.

3. Hormonal: Headaches are cyclic, usually before the menstrual period. This can also be caused by anemia and low iron stores. High estrogen and low progesterone around day 18 lead to headaches and could require the addition of supplemental progesterones.

4. Hypertensive: Found to be related to high blood pressure.

5. Food allergy: Wheat is the most common food to cause headaches followed by dairy and corn.

6. Constipation: The blood becomes toxic because of absorbed toxins from fecal waste sitting too long in the body.

7. Dehydration: Low water intake combined with too much coffee (a natural diuretic) makes the blood too concentrated.

8. Excess sleep: Too much rest and sleeping outside the normal body rhythms can cause headaches.

9. Low blood sugar: Eating refined carbohydrates spikes insulin, causing a drop in blood sugar several hours later. One of the symptoms of low blood sugar is headaches.

10. Dental disorders: Dental mercury, chronic root canal inflammation, and poor jaw alignment can cause headaches.

After completing the seven-day detoxification program, use the following strategies to combat headaches:

- Adequate water: 3 quarts per day

- Massage to relax the muscles of the neck

- Elimination of coffee, caffeine, sugar, and alcohol

- Magnesium: 300 mg twice per day

Migraine headaches are thought to be caused by serotonin release from blood platelets. This causes a constriction in blood vessels followed by rebound vasodilation due to platelet aggregation. Food allergies, hormones, and intestinal toxicity are the most common causes of the platelets that create migraine headaches.

After completing the seven-day detoxification program, use the following strategies to combat migraines:

- Adequate water: 3 quarts per day

- Elimination of coffee, caffeine, sugar, and alcohol

- Magnesium: 300 mg twice per day

- Feverfew: 50 to 82 mg per day; takes 4 to 6 weeks to work. For acute attacks, 1,000 to 2,000 mg. Feverfew prevents degranulation of platelets and thus decreases serotonin release. If feverfew isn't working, follow up with ginkgo, which inhibits platelet aggregation factor.

- Vitamin B_2: 400 mg per day with breakfast

For acute migraines, try the following:

- Meyer's intravenous magnesium injection.

For weight loss, try the following:

- Avoid food allergies.

- Make sure there is no "occult" hypothyroidism.

- Take no carbohydrates at your evening meal.

- Avoid all snacks, and eat only three meals per day.

- Shoot for losing 1 pound per week after doing the seven-day EcoTox program. Remember, for every 1 pound lost, this is equivalent to 3,500 calories.

- Aerobic exercise for 15 minutes three to four times a day. Maximum heart rate level is 220 minus age. Ideally, you want to achieve 60 to 85 percent of maximum rate (usually 120 to 160).

- Do not go on a diet providing fewer than 1,500 calories per day.

- Take 300 mg of Guggulipid three times per day.

APPENDIX D:
HOW TO
REACH US

Dr. Bennett's office can be reached at 250-544-4331. Dr. Barrie is unavailable for professional consultations at this time.

Nutritional Products

For information on nutritional detoxification products, phone 1-866-77-DETOX (1-866-773-3869) toll free or read the notes below on supplements.

Health Retreats

For information on rejuvenation health retreats, visit Dr. Bennett's Web site at www.peterbennett.com or call his office.

Personal Consultations

For information on private consultations with Dr. Bennett, phone his office or log on to his Web site.

Finding a Practitioner

Find a doctor who is willing to help you use the strategies outlined in this book. He or she might be a medical doctor, a chiropractor, or a naturopathic physician and might also be a trained nutritionist or wellness counselor. The health care practitioner that you consult might already use a detoxification program that does not exactly fit the format laid out in this book. If you feel that this doctor has a good understanding of your case and has had good results using a program that is similar to ours, always trust the application of detoxification strategies that are unique to him.

Below is a list of professional organizations that can help you find a qualified practitioner in your area:

Institute for Functional Medicine: Trains doctors to use detoxification medicine. 800-228-0622, Web site:www.fxmed.com

American Association of Naturopathic Physicians (AANP): Professional organization of naturopathic physicians. 703-610-9037, Web site: www.naturopathic.com

Canadian Naturopathic Association (CNA): 416-496-8633 www.naturopathicassoc.ca

Finding Nutritional Supplements

Many people have called us to say that it was difficult to find the supplements that they needed in health food stores. To help with this problem, we have several recommendations:

1. Contact a Quixtar or Nutrilite independent business owner in your area to locate a distributor of Nutralite supplements, which are manufactured by Amway. Or you can contact the Better Life Institute (at www.blionline.com or call 616-776-6490) and ask them to supply you with a basic package. All of their supplements have an excellent proprietary blend of bioflavonoids and plant concentrates to provide extra protection from free-radical and oxidative damage. Quixtar is a sister company of Alticor, Inc. in Ada, Michigan, and Nutrilite brand of products is distributed by Quixtar. This would include:

   • Double X: A high-potency phytonutrient vitamin and mineral supplement

   • Milk thistle, dandelion, and turmeric

   • Antioxidant complex with pycnogenol and/or grape seed extract

   • Protein powder

2. Contact a local holistic physician (M.D., N.D., D.C., or D.O.) who has experience in detoxification medicine and ask that he or she guide you and supply you with the necessary nutritional supplements.

3. Contact my office (250-544-4331) and ask for a drop ship to your door.

4. Work with a natural health food store or pharmacy to find the items you need.

   The core supplement program that you will need consists of four items:

A multivitamin with trace minerals

A powerful antioxidant (alpha lipoic acid, curcumin, vitamin E, or vitamin C)

An herb combination to protect the liver

A rice protein powder

NOTES

Detoxification Annotated Reading List
by Subject

This is a technical section for those interested in the scientific basis of detoxification medicine. Please note that medical definitions are not given because of the depth of some of the biochemical concepts. The citations and summaries here are presented as information assembled for those who want an in-depth review of detoxification. This review of medical literature is only a small sampling of material that exists on many of these subjects. Common topics that are easily referenced in popular nutritional literature are only briefly referenced and not reviewed with commentary. Those articles that I found that provided compelling information are reviewed. As a disclaimer, many times the review that I provide has to do with what I found interesting rather than what you may really need to know.

I am indebted to Jeff Bland, Ph.D., at Healthcomm Inc. in Gig Harbor, Washington, for bringing many of these articles to my attention.

Acidophilus

Kennedy, R.J., S.J. Kirk, and K.R. Gardiner. "Promotion of a Favorable Gut Flora in Inflammatory Bowel Disease." *J Parenter Enteral Nutr* 24, 3 (2000): 189–95.

This article highlights the strategy of establishing proper microbial balance in the gut environment, an important and powerful method of treating and preventing inflammatory bowel disease (IBD). The conclusions of this study present strong evidence that both Crohn's disease and ulcerative colitis, the two main forms of IBD, often develop and progress as microbe populations in the gut become imbalanced. "There is evidence that IBD patients have altered concentrations of bacteria in their feces and associated with their intestinal mucosa," the reviewers report. Low levels of protective bacteria such as *Lactobacillus* and *Bifidobacteria* in IBD patients can lead to the overgrowth of gut pathogens such as the anaerobic microbes *Bacteroides* and invasive *E. coli* associated with more severe disease symptoms. Adequate amounts of good bacteria keep potential gut pathogens in check by promoting a more acidic environment hostile to pathogen growth and by providing fuel for the cells that line the intestine, helping to keep the gut barrier intact and healthy. By sticking to the intestinal wall, friendly microbes also block the adherence and overgrowth of pathogens and help boost local gut immune function.

Modern changes in diet, however, including increased use of food preservatives and overconsumption of refined carbohydrates, can throw the natural balance of gut microbes in the human body out of whack. Crohn's disease was virtually unknown in pre-twentieth-century times and is still uncommon in rural areas of nonindustrialized countries.

A dual therapy that uses a synergistic combination of prebiotics, the ingestion of foodstuffs that promote growth of beneficial gut microbes, and probiotics (oral supplementation with live microbial cultures) is emerging as a promising treatment modality for optimizing gut flora balance in patients with IBD.

Lee, Y.K., and S. Salminen. "The Coming Age of Probiotics," *Trends Food Sci Technol* 6 (1995): 241–45.

Friend, B.A., and K.M. Shahani. "Nutritional and Therapeutic Aspects of Lactobacilli," *J Appl Nutr* 36 (1984): 125–36.

The following article summaries on *Lactobacillus* have been modified with permission from ITServices - www.clinicalpearls.com.

Lidbeck, A., and C.E. Nord. "Lactobacilli in Relation to Human Ecology and Antimicrobial Therapy," *Int J Tissue React* 8, 2 (1991): 115–22.

Lactobacilli is a therapeutic agent in the normalization of intestinal flora. Antibiotic therapy is the most common cause for altering intestinal microflora. *Lactobacillus* supplementation after antibiotic therapy to normalize intestinal flora has had mixed results in the literature.

Drutz, David J. "Lactobacillus Prophylaxis for Candida Vaginitis," *Ann Intern Med* 116, 5 (1992): 419–20.

Lactobacillus acidophilus displaces candida normally residing in the gastrointestinal tract, thereby reducing the opportunity for autoinoculation of the vagina from the perianal area and perineum.

Truss, C. Orian, et al. "Generalized Symptoms in Women with Chronic Yeast Vaginitis: Treatment with Nystatin, Diet, and Immunotherapy Versus Nystatin Alone," *J Adv Med* 5, 3 (1992): 139–75.

This study concludes that superficial yeast infection may lead to generalized symptoms and that a therapeutic six-week trial of nystatin, diet, and immunotherapy is an inexpensive way of identifying whether the yeast is the cause of the symptoms. It was noted that symptoms of chronic fatigue syndrome are closely related to this superficial candidiasis syndrome.

Aflatoxins

Ghadirian, P., et al. "Food Habits and Esophageal Cancer: An Overview," *Cancer Prev Detect* 16 (1992): 163–68.

Ames, B.N. "Dietary Carcinogens and Anticarcinogen: Oxygen Radicals and Degenerative Disease," *Science* 221, 4616 (1983): 1256–64.

Murray, R., et al. *Harper's Biochemistry.* Norwalk, CT: Appleton and Lange, 1993.

Manahan, S.E. *Toxicological Chemistry.* Chelsea, MI: Lewis Publishers, 1992.

Aging

Lipsitz, L.A., and A.L. Goldberger. "Loss of Complexity and Aging," *JAMA* 267, 13 (1992): 1806–9.

Aging relates to the breakdown of organ complexity and functional reserve. Fractals and chaos may provide ways to measure aging. An example in physiology is the branching architecture of anatomy, including nerve networks, His-Purkinje fibers, GI folding (rugae), and vascular systems.

Chaos describes unpredictable behavior that may arise from internal feedback loops of nonlinear systems such as constrained randomness of the heartbeat in healthy individuals. As an example of chaos related to human health, despite the nearly identical mean and standard deviation for a young man's and old man's heartbeat, the complexity signal is markedly reduced in an older subject.

Similarly, fractals are used in wellness assessment. Fractals do not have a single characteristic scale of length, and chaos does not have a characteristic scale of time. Loss of complexity (aging) is accompanied by narrowing in random structure (fractals) and rhythm (chaos) of organs. Detoxification medicine seeks to preserve the complexity of physiological functioning through optimum performance.

Air Quality

Ross, C.P., J.S. Ross, and K. Asseiro. "Sick Building Syndrome," *J Orthomol Med* 12, 1 (1997): 23–28.

Alcohol

Lieber, C.S. "Alcohol, Liver and Nutrition," *J Am Coll Nutr* 10, 6 (1991): 602–32.

Changes are linked to redox changes produced by reduced nicotinamide adenine dinucleotide (NAD) generated via alcohol dehydrogenase pathway. Ethanol can be oxidized by a microsomal oxidizing system involving cyp450. The newly discovered ethanol inducible cytochrome (P-450 IIE1) contributes to ethanol metabolism tolerance, energy wastage, and selective perivenular toxicity of various xenobiotics.

Aluminum

Rifat, S. "Aluminum Hypothesis Lives," *Lancet* 336 (1990): 1162–65.

White, D.M., et al. "Neurologic Syndrome in 25 Workers from an Aluminum Smelting Plant," *Arch Intern Med* 152 (1992): 1443–48.

Knoll, O., et al. "Consequences from EEG Findings and Aluminum Encephalopathy," *Trace Element Med* 8 (1991): S18–20.

Ancient Methods of Detoxification

Johns, T. DuQuette. "Detoxification and Mineral Supplementation as Functions of Geophagy," *Am J Clin Nutr* 53 (1991): 448–56.

The use of clay as a primitive detoxification substance is presented.

Antioxidants

Bland, J.S. "Oxidants and Antioxidants in Clinical Medicine: Past, Present and Future Potential," *J Nutr Environ Med* 5 (1995): 255–80.

Thorough and complete review of the historical and biochemical landmarks of antioxidant biochemistry.

Aust, S.D., C.F. Chignell, T.M. Bray, et al. "Free Radicals in Toxicology," *Toxicol Appl Pharmacol* 120 (1993): 68–178.

Stocker, R., et al. "Endogenous Antioxidant Defenses in Human Blood Plasma." In Sies, H., ed. *Oxidative Stress.* New York: Academic Press, 1985: 224–25.

Asthma

Hamilton, K. *Asthma: Clinical Pearls in Nutrition and Complementary Therapies.* Sacramento, CA: IT Services, 1997.

Comprehensive review of medical literature on the causes and treatment of asthma.

"The Increasing Burden of Asthma in the Young," *Morbidity and Mortality Weekly Report* 45, 17 (1996): 350–53.

Rennick, G.J., and F.C. Jarman. "Are Children with Asthma Affected by Smog?" *Med J Australia* 156 (1992): 837–41.

Burr, M.L. "Pollution: Does It Cause Asthma?" *Arch Dis Child* 72 (1995): 377–87.

Barley Extract

Kitta, K., et al. "Antioxidant Activity of an Isoflavonoid 2-glycosylisovitexin (2-O-GIV) Isolated from Green Barley Leaves," *J Agric Food Chem* 40 (1992): 1843–45.

Betaine

Barak, A.J., et al. "Betaine, Ethanol, and the Liver: A Review," *Alcohol* 13, 4 (1996): 395–98.

Wilcken, D.E., B. Wilckin, and N.P. Dudman, et al. "Homocysteineuria: The Effects of Betaine in the Treatment of Patients Not Responsive to Pyridoxine," *NEJM* 309, 8 (1983): 448–53.

Bile Salts

Schoenfield, L.J., et al. "Chenodiol (Chenodoxycholic Acid) for Dissolution of Gallstones. The National Cooperative Gallstone Study," *Ann Intern Med* 95 (1981): 257.

Cancer

Steingraber, S. *Living Downstream: An Ecologist Looks At Cancer and the Environment.* Reading, MA: Addison-Wesley, 1997.

A must read review of the environmental impact of pesticides.

Ries, L.A., et al. "SEER Cancer Statistics Review, 1971–1991: Tables and Graphs," NIH Pub. 94-2789 (Bethesda, MD: NCI, 1994): 428.

Raloff, J. "Ecocancers: Do Environmental Factors Underlie a Breast Cancer Epidemic?" *Sci News* 144 (1993): 10–13.

An unintended side effect of industrialization may be an environment that bathes its inhabitants in a sea of pollutants with estrogenic effects.

Epstein, S.S. *Politics of Cancer.* San Francisco, CA: Sierra Club Books, 1978.

Charcoal

Roberts, J.R., E.J. Gracely, et al. "Advantage of High Surface Area Charcoal for Gastrointestinal Decontamination in a Human Acetominophen Ingestion Model," *Acad Emerg Med* 4 (1997): 167–74.

Thrash, A., and C. Thrash. *Home Remedies.* Seale, AL: Thrash Publications, 1981.

Chewing Food

Playford, R.J., et al. "Effect of Luminal Growth Factor Preservation on Intestinal Growth," *Lancet* 341 (1993): 843–50.

Chewing stimulates the secretion of a growth factor that prevents intestinal permeability.

Children and Toxins

Raloff, J. "Breast Milk: A Leading Source of PCBs," *Sci News* 152 (1997): 344.

173 children who were breast fed carried some trace of PCBs in their blood by age 42 months. This gives them 3.6 times higher levels than formula-fed babies. PCBs diminish a child's ability to learn.

Savits, D. "Home Pesticide Use and Childhood Cancer: A Case Control Study," *Am J Public Health* 249 (1995): 249–52.

Seppa, N. "Exposure to Smoke Yields Fetal Mutations," *Sci News* 154 (1998): 213.

Some studies have associated pregnant mothers' exposure to tobacco smoke with increased incidence of childhood leukemia and lymphoma. Because pediatric tumors occur early, the genetic changes associated with them may start in the womb with the mutation of genes (HRPT) causing the misguided action of DNA repair enzymes.

Fackelman, K.A. "Dad's Farming May Hike Baby's Liver Risk," *Sci News* 140 (1991): 6.

Pesticides can induce rare liver disorders in unborn children.

"Organochlorines Lace Inuit Breast Milk," *Sci News* (12 February 1994): 111.

Inuit Indians eat seal and whale blubber laced with DDT, and it shows up in the breast milk. High concentrations of omega-3 fatty acids in the diet probably protect the infants from neurological damage.

"Pesticides in Produce May Threaten Kids," *Sci News* 144 (1993): 4–5.

Estimates that one-third of a child's lifetime exposure to pesticides will accumulate by age 5. By the child's first birthday, exposure to carcinogenic pesticides will exceed the federal government's lifetime acceptable cancer-risk threshold calculated to result in one malignancy in every million individuals.

Chronic Fatigue/Fibromyalgia/Chemical Sensitivity

Rigden, S. "Entero-Hepatic Resuscitation Program for CIFIDS," *The CIFIDS Chronicle* (Spring 1995): 46–49.

Arnold, D.I., et al. "Excessive Intracellular Acidosis of Skeletal Muscle on Exercise in a Patient with Post Viral Exhaustion/Fatigue Syndrome," *Lancet* 1 (1984): 1367–68.

Mukherji, T.M., et al. "Abnormal Red Blood Cell Morphology in Myalgic Encephalomyelitis," *Lancet* 2 (1987): 328–29.

Buchwald, D., and D. Garrity. "Comparison of Patients with Chronic Fatigue Syndrome, Fibromyalgia and Multiple Chemical Sensitivities," *Arch Intern Med* 154 (1994): 2049–53.

Buist, R.A. "Chronic Fatigue Syndrome and Chemical Overload," *Int Clin Nutr Rev* 8, 4 (1988): 173–75.

Chronic Disease

Glazier, W.H. "The Task of Medicine," *Sci Am* 228, 4 (1973): 13–18.

A summary of the transition in medicine from treating acute disease as the main cause of death at the turn of the century to treating chronic degenerative disease as we enter the second millennium. It points to the need of physicians to acquire skills necessary for this trend rather than relying on "heroic" methods.

Constipation

Iacono, G., et al. "Chronic Constipation as a Symptom of Cow's Milk Allergy," *J Pediatr* 126 (1995): 34–39.

Dehydration and Toxicity

Wills, M. "Uremic Toxins and Their Effects on Intermediary Metabolism," *Clin Chem* 13, 1 (1985): 5–13.

Uremia is a manifestation of a wide variety of disorders. The retention of metabolic end products and their effects as toxins act on intermediary metabolism. At the cell membrane level, the action occurs. No one individual compound has been implicated as the uremic toxin.

Diet

Bland, J.,S., E. Barringer, R.G. Reedy, and K. Bland. "A Medical
Food Supplemented Detoxification Program in the Management of Chronic Health Problems," *Altern Ther* 1, 5 (1995):
62–71.

Original research documenting the effectiveness of medical
detoxification programs for treating chronic health problems.

Simopoulos, A.P. "Diet and Gene Interactions," *Food Tech* 51, 3
(1997): 66–69.

Using the tools of molecular biology and genetics, research is
defining the mechanisms by which genes influence nutrient absorption, metabolism, and excretion, taste perception, degree of
satiation, and the mechanisms by which nutrients influence gene
expression.

Endotoxins

Editorial. "Intestinal Endotoxins as Mediators of Hepatic Injury:
An Idea Whose Time Has Come Again," *Hepatology* 10, 5
(1989): 881–91.

The concept of "autointoxication" has resurfaced from the nineteenth century as endotoxins. Endotoxins are the lipopolysac-
caride (LPS) outer walls of gram-negative bacteria that have died.
This macromolecule can transit the gut. Endotoxemia has gained
favor as an explanation for the multiple organ failure with severe
trauma and sepsis. Endotoxemia is associated with Crohn's and
neonatal enterocolitis. Animals that are induced to fatty liver degeneration are exquisitely sensitive to LPS injection where controls are not. Integrity of detoxification and immune system is
critical in the response to endotoxins. Complications in chronic
liver disease can be induced by LPS. LPS is scavenged by Kupffer
cells; this then depresses p450 and impairs mitochondrial function. Strong injurious products are released by macrophages exposed to LPS, causing the need for antioxidants. Alcohol is known
to aggravate LPS toxicity.

Environmental Health

Beasley, J., and J. Swift, eds. *The Kellogg Report: The Impact of Nutrition, Environment and Lifestyle on the Health of Americans.* Annandale-on-Hudson, NY: The Institute of Health Policy and Practice, The Bard College Center, 1989.

Remarkable overview of the impact on society by American lifestyle and industry. Thorough and readable.

Manahan, S.E. *Toxicological Chemistry.* Chelsea, MI: Lewis Publishers, 1992.

Steingraber, S. *Living Downstream: An Ecologist Looks at Cancer and the Environment.* Reading, MA: Addison-Wesley, 1997.

U.S. Environmental Protection Agency. *1987–1994 Toxic Release Inventory National Report.* Washington, DC: Office of Toxic Substances, 1994.

"A Two Decade Drop in Sperm Counts." *Sci News* (25 February 1995): 127.

Dougherty, R.C., et al. "Negative Chemical Ionization Studies of Human and Food Chain Contamination with Xenobiotic Chemicals," *Environ Health Perspect* 36 (1980): 103–17.

Bertram, H.P., et al. "Hexachlorobenzene Content in Human Whole Blood and Adipose Tissue: Experiences in Environmental Specimen Banking," *IARC Sci Pub* 77 (1986): 173–82.

Estrogen, Xenoestrogens, Estrogen Mimicking, and Detoxification

Begley, S., and D. Glick. "The Estrogen Complex," *Newsweek* (21 March 1994): 76–77.

Musey, P.I., et al. "Effect of Diet on Oxidation of 17 Beta Estradiol in Vivo," *J Clin Endocrinol Metab* 65 (1987): 792–95.

Rohan, T.E., et al. "Diet in the Etiology of Breast Cancer," *Epidemiology* 9 (1987): 120–45.

Hershoff, R.J., and H.L. Bradlow. "Obesity, Diet, Endogenous Estrogens, and the Risk of Hormone Sensitive Cancer," *Am J Clin Nutr* 45 (1987): 283–89.

Schneider, J., et al. "Effects of Obesity on Estradiol Metabolism: Decreased Formation of Nonuterotropic Metabolites," *J Clin Endocrinol Metab* 56 (1983): 973–78.

Ralaoff, J. "Beyond Estrogens: Why Unmasking Hormone-Mimicking Pollutants Proves so Challenging," *Sci News* 148 (1995): 44–45.

Steingraber, S. *Living Downstream: An Ecologist Looks at Cancer and the Environment.* Reading, MA: Addison-Wesley, 1997.

Raloff, J. "Lacing Food with an Estrogen Mimic," *Sci News* 152 (1997): 255.

Bisphenol is well known to produce estrogen mimicking. This article shows that the building block of polycarbonate plastics, bisphenol A, is found in food that is heated in plastic. Polycarbonate plastics are made by linking bisphenol A into long chains. Not every molecule gets linked or polymerized, leaving free product to migrate from the finished product. In tests by the FDA, results show that bisphenol can leach into liquids. Polycarbonate baby bottles and juice caps contained up to 46 micrograms of unbound bisphenol A per gram of plastic.

Raloff, J. "Plastics May Shed Chemical Estrogens," *Sci News* 144 (1993): 12.

Bisphenol A from polycarbonate food containers is able to exhibit hormonal activity at concentrations of just 2 to 5 parts per billion. On the other hand, plastics are considered safe if they shed 10 parts per billion.

Raloff, J. "That Feminine Touch: Are Men Suffering from Prenatal or Childhood Exposure to 'Hormonal' Toxicants?" *Sci News* 145 (1994): 56–58.

A single peach can carry residues of up to six pesticides. These pesticides effect the activity of the testicles. There is an increased trend toward hormone-related problems like undescended testicles, testicular cancer (tripled in the last 50 years), and falling sperm counts. We must ask the question whether there can be an economic cost put on having a generation that cannot reproduce because of chemical estrogens.

Noteboom, W.D., and J. Gorski. "Estrogenic Effect of Genistein and Coumestrol Diacetate. *Endocrinology* 73 (1963): 736–39.

Plants have estrogenic effects. (These might be used to block the effects of xenoestrogens from the environment.)

Raloff, J. "The Gender Benders: Are Environmental 'Hormones' Emasculating Wildlife?" *Sci News* 145 (1996): 24–27.

DDT, PCBs, kepone, heptachlor, dieldrin, mirex, and toxaphene exhibit properties of "environmental hormones," mimicking the effects of naturally produced hormones such as estrogen. This fact may be contributing to reproductive cancers in females. Animal data suggest that far smaller exposures to these substances are needed to trigger reproductive effects than to produce cancers. Because these reproductive changes may be subtle, they could evade detection for decades.

"Gender-Bending PCBs," *Sci News* (8 October 1994): 239.

PCBs can alter gender in animals, turning males into females at very small doses.

Farming

Hall, R.H. *Food for Naught: The Decline in Nutrition.* New York: Random House/Vintage Books, 1976.

Gibons, B. "Do We Treat Our Soil Like Dirt?" *National Geographic* 166, 3 (1984): 350–88.

Fasting

Lee, C., et al. "Age Associated Alterations of the Mitochondrial Genome," *Free Radic Biol Med* 22, 7 (1997): 1259–69.

Oxygen destroys mitochondrial genomes that lack DNA repair mechanisms. Diet restriction (fasting) is the only consistently proven method of extending life span, and this article hypothesizes that it is because it reduces the total amount of oxidative stress within an animal. Diet restriction can attenuate age-associated mitochondrial enzymatic dysfunction.

Vogt, B.L., and J.P. Ritchie. "Fasting-Induced Depletion of Glutathione in the Aging Mouse," *Biochem Pharmacol* 46, 2 (1993): 257–63.

Boyd, E.M., and F.L. Taylor. "The Acute Oral Toxicity of Chlordane in Albino Rats Fed for 28 Days from Weaning on a Protein-Deficient Diet," *Input Med Surg* 1 (1969): 213–51.

Godin, D.V., and S.A. Wohaier. "Nutritional Deficiency, Starvation and Tissue Antioxidant Status," *Free Radic Biol Med* 5 (1988): 165–76.

Low tissue antioxidant status is found under dietary restriction. Free-radical pathology is usually involved in toxicity and diseases like diabetes, cancer, and atherosclerosis. Nutritional deficiencies change specific antioxidant enzymes: Se, Cu, Mn, Zn, vitamin E, vitamin B_2, vitamin C, and sulfur amino acids are all needed for detoxification. Fasting alters glutathione-dependent detoxification, the practice of fasting a patient and then putting him or her through chemical exposure like an anesthetic places them at risk. Patients who will undergo surgery would probably have less complications to the anesthetic if they were put on a nutrient-dense regimen.

Chaitow, L. "Fasting and Detoxification," *J Alt Compll Med* 14, 3 (March 1996).

Food Allergies

Hunter, J.O. "Food Allergy or Enterometabolic Disorder," *Lancet* 338 (1991): 495–96.

Allergies from foods are multifactorial in causes. A single mechanism by which patients react to foods is at present unclear.

Historically, diets are found to be useful in migraine headaches, irritable bowel syndrome (IBS), Crohn's disease, eczema, hyperactivity, and rheumatoid arthritis. Because there are occasionally no findings in the IgE and RAST (radioallergoabsorbent testing), such results lead some investigators to conclude that food allergy symptoms are merely neurotic symptoms.

Inhibitors of detoxification might be coming from gut flora. We know that encephalopathy in cirrhotic patients develops after a meal where they cannot metabolize the amino compounds produced by gut flora. The gut produces a wide array of substances that cause reactions with all organs in the body. Colonic microflora produce a wide variety of chemicals; in susceptible individuals with reduced hepatic enzymes, they pass into systemic circulation to produce symptoms at distant parts. It is well known that IBS can come on after surgery, radiation, gastroenteritis, and the use of antibiotics, all of which may change the bowel flora. Levels of facultative anaerobes rise after a food challenge in patients with IBS. Food allergy may not be an immunologic disease but a disorder of bacterial fermentation and enzyme deficiency. Enteroadherent *E. coli* are present in the stool in a high percentage of patients with a variety of food-related autoimmune problems such as Crohn's disease. Abnormal bacteria are also found in patients with RA, ankylosing spondylitis. HLA B_{27} is synthesized by the fecal flora and associated with the facultative anaerobes klebsiella and proteus.

Foods have their own reactions that they generate outside of allergy models. For example, tyramine in chocolate causes bouts of headaches in susceptible people because of a genetic inability to detoxify this vasoactive amine before it goes out into systemic circulation. This is probably related to genetic predisposition; patients with migraines have a low level of monoamine oxidase (MAO) and phenolsulphotransferase (PST).

Scadding, G.K., et al. "Poor Sulfoxidation Ability in Patients with Food Sensitivity," *Br Med J* 297 (1988): 105–7.

Van Hooser, B., and L.V.C. Crawford. "Allergy Diets for Infants and Children," *Comprehen Ther* 15 (1989): 38–47.

Cordle, C.T. "Control of Food Allergies Using Protein Hydrolysates," *Food Technol* (October 1994): 72–76.

Dockhorn, R.J., and T.C. Smith. "Use of Chemically Defined Hypoallergenic Diet (Vivonex®) in the Management of Patients with Suspected Food Allergy/Intolerance," *Ann Allergy* 47 (1981): 264–66.

Miller, S.B. "IgG Food Allergy Testing by ELISA/EIA: What Do They Really Tell Us?" *Townsend Lett Doctors Patients* 174 (1998): 62–65.

The use of a food allergy tests does not preclude the use of an elimination diet for treatment of food allergies or more accurately determine the nature of what J.O. Hunter calls "enterometabolic disorders."

Rafei, A.E., et al. "The Diagnostic Value of IgG$_4$ Measurements in Patients with Food Allergy." *Ann Allergy* 62 (1989): 94–99.

Metcalfe, D.D. "The Nature and Mechanism of Food Allergies and Related Diseases," *Food Technol* (May 1992): 136–39.

The author feels that food shouldn't be attributed to diseases and symptoms because he can't find a scientific basis for the reactions. He should probably read the article by J.O. Hunter above. The author does provide a good review on the subject of food allergies. There are three types: IgE, immune complex, and delayed hypersensitivity.

Achlorhydria, cystic fibrosis, selective IgA deficiency, or gastrointestinal immaturity lead to increased penetration of the gut barrier by antigens. Alcohol, aspirin, and tobacco may reduce gastric mucus and thereby contribute to the disruption of the epithelial barrier. Factors that affect the amount of antigen absorbed include the amount of antigen ingested, whether the antigen was consumed with other foods, the degree of cooking that renders proteins more soluble, and gastrointestinal inflammation. It has been demonstrated that food proteins penetrate even normal gastrointestinal tracts. Gluten sensitivity is a delayed reaction. Abdominal pain, vomiting, diarrhea, and failure to thrive are the symptoms in children with food allergies.

The immunopathology of these disorders is not completely understood. There may be more than one immune-mediated mechanism at work.

McCabe, B.J. "Dietary Tyramine and Other Pressor Amines in MAOI Regimens: A Review," *J Am Diet Assoc* 86 (1986): 1059–64.

Madara, J.L. "Pathobiology of the Intestinal Epithelial Barrier," *Am J Pathol* 137, 6 (1990): 1273–81.

Madsen, C. "Prevalence of Food Additive Intolerance," *Hum Exp Toxicol* 13 (1994): 393–99.

Pennisi, E. "Food Allergies Linked to Ear Infections," *Sci News* 146 (1994): 231.

Ogle, K.A., and J.D. Bullock. "Children with Allergic Rhinitis and/or Bronchial Asthma Treated with Elimination Diet: A Five Year Follow-Up," *Ann Allergy* 44 (1980): 273–78.

Food and Nutrient Levels

Smith, B. "Organic Foods Versus Supermarket Foods: Element Levels," *J Appl Nutr* 45 (1993): 35–39.

Food and Water Contamination

Steingraber, S. *Living Downstream: An Ecologist Looks at Cancer and the Environment.* Reading, MA: Addison-Wesley, 1997.

Beasley, J., and J. Swift, eds. *The Kellogg Report: The Impact of Nutrition, Environment and Lifestyle on the Health of Americans.* Annandale-on-Hudson, NY: The Institute of Health Policy and Practice, The Bard College Center, 1989.

California Department of Consumer Affairs. "Clean Your Room: A Compendium on Indoor Pollution," Sacramento, 1982 (cited in *The Kellogg Report*, page 175).

Food Toxins

Roberts, P.R., and G.P. Zaloga. "Dietary Bioactive Peptides," *New Horizons* 2, 2 (1994): 237–43.

Gaitan, E., et al. "In Vitro Measurement of Antithyroid Compounds and Environmental Goitrogens," *J Clin Endocrinol Metab* 56 (1983): 767–73.

Raloff, J. "How Cooked Meat May Inflame the Heart," *Sci News* 145 (1994): 145.

Formaldehyde

Main, D.M., and T.J. Hogan. "Health Effects of Low-Level Exposures to Formaldehyde," *J Occup Med* 25 (1983): 896–900.

Graefstrom, R.C., A.J. Fornore, H. Autrop, et al. "Formaldehyde Damage to DNA and Inhibition of DNA Repair in Human Bronchial Cells," *Science* 220 (1982): 216–17.

Ross, C.P., J.S. Ross, and K. Asseiro. "Sick Building Syndrome," *J Orthomol Med* 12, 1 (1997): 23–28.

Bardana, E. "Formaldehyde," *Immunol Allergy Practice* 2, 3 (1980): 11–23.

Gallstones

Tuzhlin, S.A., et al. "The Treatment of Patients with Gallstones by Lecithin," *Am J Gastroenterol* 65 (1976): 231.

McDougall, R.M., et al. "Effect of Wheat Bran on Serum Lipoproteins and Biliary Lipids," *Can J Surg* 21 (1978): 433.

Breneman, J.C. "Allergy Elimination Diet as the Most Effective Gallbladder Diet," *Ann Allergy* 26 (1968): 83.

Genetic Susceptibility to Toxicity

McFadden, S.A. "Phenotypic Variation in Xenobiotic Metabolism and Adverse Environmental Response: Focus on Sulfur-Dependent Detoxification Pathways," *Toxicology* 111 (1996): 43–65.

Excellent review of detoxification pathways from the standpoint of ecogenetic polymorphisms.

Variations in sulfation and sulfoxidation are inherited metabolic polymorphisms. A significant number of individuals with environmental intolerance or chronic disease have impaired sulfation of phenolic substances from starvation of sulfotransferases for sulfate substrate. Sulfation is a limited capacity xenobiotic conjugation pathway that is present in many tissues. Impaired sulfation may be relevant to intolerance to phenol, tyramine, and phenolic food constituents. This biochemical pathway may be the link to explaining Dr. B. Feingold's (*Why Your Child Is Hyperactive*, New York: Random House, 1975) findings that some children react to food colorings and preservatives. This represents a unique consideration of treatment of depletion/disruption of sulfate pool in diet-responsive Feingold patients, autistics. Depletion of sulfates might elevate endogenous biocomponents like bile acids and joint glucosamine glycans and primary biliary cirrhosis and rheumatoid arthritis. The sulfate conjugation of phenolics is an important pathway for the detoxification of catecholamine neurotransmitters, steroids, bile acids, phenolic and aromatic drugs, and xenobiotics. Impaired sulfation may cause tyramine headache and poor first-pass sulfation of monoamines. Tyramine is a bacterial fermentation product closely related to catecholamine neurotransmitters, found in cheese, wine, and so on.

Examples of diseases with genetically influenced reduced sulfoxidation (SO), reduced sulfation (S), and elevated cysteine and sulfate ratio (Cys/So4) include:

- Alzheimer's disease—Reduced SO, S, Cys/So4

- Parkinson's disease—Reduced SO, S, Cys/So4

- Motor neuron disease—Reduced SO, S, Cys/So4

- Autism—Reduced SO, S, Cys/So4

- Systemic lupus erythematosus—Reduced SO, Cys/So4

- Primary biliary cirrhosis—Reduced SO, Cys/So4

- Rheumatoid arthritis—Reduced SO, S, Cys/So4

- Chlorpromazine jaundice—Reduced SO

- D-penicillamine toxicity in rheumatoid arthritis—Reduced SO

- Non IgE food sensitivity—Reduced SO

- Multiple chemical sensitivity—Reduced SO

Reading, C. "Family Tree Connection: How Your Past Can Shape Your Future Health: A Lesson in Orthomolecular Medicine," *J Orthomol Med* 3, 3 (1988): 123–34.

Christopher Reading, M.D., has evaluated the case histories of over 5,000 patients and strongly advises doctors and patients to draw up family trees showing diagnosed illnesses. He discovered that it is extremely important to draw up a family tree. It is important to study the various ways certain genetic disorders are inherited. For example, a father cannot pass on an X-linked disorder to his son because his son only gets the Y chromosome from his father but all the daughters are at risk. Dr. Reading found one family where the manic depression was X linked with an additional X-linked B_{12} deficiency. The B_{12} deficiency was later found to be due to wheat allergies, a common inherited trait. He treated this family with vitamin B_{12} and a gluten-free diet. Their anemia and manic depression resolved.

Daly, A.K., S. Cholerton, W. Gregory, and J.R. Idle. "Metabolic Polymorphisms," *Pharmacol Ther* 57 (1993): 129–60.

There is a wide array of genotypic and phenotypic polymorphisms of xenobiotic metabolizing enzymes. P450 variations represent the best studied group of xenobiotic enzymes. There is a wide variety in how people can metabolize drugs and different drug groups. Drug reactions cause 30 percent of hospital admissions. If more testing was done, more diseases like cancer susceptibility (glutathione-s-transferase and lung cancer) and polymorphisms would be better understood. For example, Parkinson's disease shows variation in CYP2D6 and breakdown of neurotoxin 1-methyl-4-phenyl-1,2,3,4-tetrahydroisoquinolne, which induces Parkinson's in certain animal species due to this p450 enzyme polymorphism.

Kaprio, J. "Science, Medicine, and the Future: Genetic Epidemiology." *Br Med J* 320, 7244 (2000):1257–59.

Research in the cause of disease has shifted toward investigating genetic causes. Genetic epidemiology has permitted identification of genes affecting people's susceptibility to disease, although progress has been much slower than many people expected. Although the role of genetic factors in diseases such as hypertension, asthma, and depression is being intensively studied, family studies and the large geographical and temporal variation in the occurrence of many diseases indicate a major role of the environment. Thus, it is necessary to consider findings about susceptibility genes in the context of a population and to evaluate the role of genetic factors in relation to other environmental factors.

Dolara, P., et al. "Urinary 6-beta-OH-cortisol and Paracetamol Metabolites as a Probe for Assessing Oxidation and Conjugation of Chemicals Inhuman," *Pharm Res Comm* 19, 4 (1987): 261–73.

There is a wide range of variation of inducers of detox enzymes in human populations.

Williams, A.C., G.B. Steventon, and R.H. Waring. "Hereditary Variation of Liver Enzymes Involved with Detoxification and Neurodegenerative Disease," *J Inherit Metab Dis* 14 (1991): 431–35.

Sonia, M.F., et al. "Decreased Glucuronidation and Increased Bioactivation of Acetaminophen in Gilbert's Syndrome," *Gastroenterology* 102 (1992): 577–86.

Mitchell, S.C., R.H. Waring, D. Land, and W.V. Thorpe. "Odorous Urine Following Asparagus Ingestion in Man," *Experientia* 4394 (1987): 382–83.

Daly, A.K., et al. "Metabolic Polymorphisms," *Pharm Ther* 57 (1993): 129–60.

Bishop, J.E., and M. Waldholtz. *Genome.* New York: Simon and Schuster, 1990.

Nebert, D.W., et al. "Human AH Locus Polymorphism and Cancer: Inducibility of CYP1A1 and Other Genes by Combustion Products and Dioxin," *Pharmacogenetics* 1 (1991): 68–78.

Detoxification polymorphisms relate with differences in risk of bronchogenic carcinoma caused by cigarette smoking.

Glucuronidation

Lee, J.R. "Fluoride Linked to Gilbert's Syndrome," *Cortlandt Forum* 101 (1985): 31–33.

Mulder, G.J., ed. *Conjugation Reactions in Drug Metabolism.* New York: Taylor and Francis, 1990: 52–91.

De Morais, S., et al. "Decreased Glucuronidation and Increased Bioactivation of Acetaminophen in Gilbert's Syndrome," *Gastroenterology* 102 (1992): 577–86.

Five to seven percent of the population gets jaundiced from Gilbert's syndrome (GS). They also get enhanced toxicity to acetaminophen. Acetaminophen glucuronide formation was 31 percent lower in GS patients. These people could have potential toxic implications for other drugs and environmental chemicals.

Aono, S., et al. "Analysis of Genes or Bilirubin UDP-glucuronsyltransferases in Gilbert's Syndrome," *Lancet* 345 (1995): 958–59.

Gilbert's syndrome is a dominant trait. Homozygotes may go on to more severe jaundice.

Glutathione

Meister, A., and M.E. Anderson. "Glutathione," *Annu Rev Biochem* 52 (1983): 711–60.

A thorough review of glutathione biochemistry.

The following article summaries on glutathione have been modified with permission from IT Services, www.clinicalpearls.com.

Julius, M. "Glutathione and Morbidity in a Community-Based Sample of Elderly," *J Clin Epidemiol* 47, 9 (1994): 1021–26.

Glutathione is a tripeptide composed of glutamic acid, cysteine, and glycine. This study indicates that ultimately medicine will regard glutathione as the body's master antioxidant and primary marker of aging. The description of biological aging, that the cell loses the ability to replicate/regenerate and the immune system declines, coincides with the major functions of glutathione in the body: protecting cells against the destructive effects of reactive oxygen intermediates and free radicals, detoxifying external substances such as drugs and environmental pollutants, maintaining cell membrane stability, regulating protein and DNA biosynthesis and cell growth, and enhancing immunologic function through its effects on lymphocytes. These widespread functions suggest that the level of glutathione has major health effects on the molecular, cellular, and organ levels of the individual. Studies have shown that there are patterns of glutathione concentrations that suggest that people who maintain high levels of glutathione, for whatever reason, represent survivors with extreme longevity. Recently, a number of small clinical studies show that with most chronic and infectious diseases, including AIDS, patients' glutathione levels are low compared to healthy controls. Conversely, high glutathione levels are being associated with good health and extreme longevity. Pine bark extract (pycnogenol), melatonin, bilberry grape extract, turmeric, and other nutrients have been shown to elevate glutathione.

Altomare, Emanuele, et al. "High-Dose Antioxidant Therapy During Thrombolysis in Patients with Acute Myocardial Infarction," *Curr Ther Res* 57, 2 (1996): 131–41.

This study evaluated 67 patients with a myocardial infarction treated with recombinant tissue-type plasminogen activator (rt-PA), of which 35 received glutathione at an intravenous bolus initially of 1,800 mg followed by $20\mu/kg$ per minute for the next 24 hours. Intravenous glutathione appears to limit the adverse effects associated with reperfusion-induced oxidative stress. If confirmed, the authors feel that glutathione administration should be considered a natural free-radical antagonist that has a high specificity and low toxicity in humans.

This study highlights the clinical fact that intravenous glutathione is a powerful way to treat many acute and chronic diseases that have oxidative damage as the cause. In my clinic, intravenous glutathione is a standard treatment for neurological diseases, cancer, cardiovascular diseases, and diseases related to toxicology.

Deledda, M.G., et al. "Reduced Intravenous Glutathione in the Treatment of Early Parkinson's Disease," *Sechi Prog Neurophyschopharmacol Biol Psychiatr* 20,7 (1996): 1159–70.

In nine patients with early, untreated Parkinson's disease, glutathione was given intravenously at 600 mg, twice daily, for 30 days in an open trial. All the patients improved significantly after glutathione therapy, with a 42 percent decline in disability. Once glutathione was stopped, the therapeutic effect lasted from 2 to 4 months. This is another research article adding to the increasing body of literature pointing to the benefit of using intravenous glutathione for a wide range of disorders.

Witschi, A., S. Reddy, B. Stofer, and B.H. Lauterburg. "The Systemic Availability of Oral Glutathione," *Eur J Clin Pharmacol* 43 (1992): 667–69.

This study points to the need of using glutathione intravenously for therapeutic effect because of the negligible effect of oral glutathione. Taking oral glutathione does not increase glutathione levels because of the hydrolysis of glutathione by intestinal and hepatic gamma-glutamyl transferase. Other oral agents besides supplemental glutathione that help maintain or elevate glutathione levels include N-acetyl-L-cysteine, lipoic acid, selenium, and vitamins E and C.

Cathcart, Robert F., III. "Glutathione and HIV Infection," *Lancet* 335 (1990): 235.

Vitamin C can be given as intravenous sodium ascorbate without preservatives at a pH of 7.0 in 60-g dosages in 500 ml of Ringer's lactate over three to four hours, one to three times daily. Ascorbate is utilized as a free-radical scavenger in these massive dosages when glutathione is exhausted and is effective in protecting glutathione levels; therefore, intravenous vitamin C should be considered a type of adjunctive glutathione therapy.

Vallis, K.A. "Glutathione Deficiency and Radiosensitivity in AIDS Patients," *Lancet* 337 (1991): 918–19.

It is known that AIDS patients have low glutathione levels. The author states that N-acetyl-L-cysteine (NAC) inhibits HIV replication, and it may do so by replenishing intracellular glutathione. It has been suggested as a beneficial therapeutic agent in AIDS, and, though untested, it may be of benefit in glutathione-deficient AIDS patients who are undergoing radiotherapy. This may help prevent some of the unwanted side effects in tissue destruction due to radiation therapy.

Bounous, G., et al. "Whey Proteins in Cancer Prevention," *Cancer Lett* 57 (1991): 91–94.

Some epidemiologic evidence suggests that dietary milk products, specifically the whey component, may have an antitumor–cancer preventive activity. Whey protein diets have been shown to increase glutathione concentrations. Whey protein is particularly rich in components needed for glutathione synthesis. The authors conclude that whey protein may have its benefits in preventing carcinogenesis by stimulating glutathione concentrations. Glutathione conjugation is a major detoxification pathway for many xenobiotics that may be potential carcinogens.

"Glutathione and Detoxification," *Cancer Treatment Rev* 17 (1990): 203–8.

The toxicity of cisplatin, an effective drug in the treatment of solid tumors, is a major problem. It is proposed in this article that glutathione is a promising antidote. Glutathione is a safe compound that prevents cisplatin-induced nephrotoxicity without affecting its antitumor activity. This would enhance the ability to use higher doses of cisplatin and improve efficacy against certain tumors. The advantage of the combination of glutathione with high doses of cisplatin was demonstrated by the impressive response rate in the treatment of ovarian cancer.

Dalhoff, K., et al. "Glutathione Treatment of Hepatocellular Carcinoma," *Liver* 12 (1992): 341–43.

Witschi, A., et al. "The Systemic Availability of Oral Glutathione," *Eur J Clin Pharmacol* 43 (1992): 667–69.

Johnston, C.J., et al. "Vitamin C Elevates Red Blood Cell Glutathione in Healthy Adults," *Am J Clin Nutr* 58 (1994): 13–105.

Burgunder, J.M., and B.H. Lauterburg. "Decreased Production of Glutathione in Patients with Cirrhosis," *Eur J Clin Invest* 17 (1987): 408–14.

The concentration of glutathione in the blood remains one of the most reliable indicators of total body glutathione, most of which is made in the liver and exported into the bloodstream.

Keterer, B., B. Coles, and D.J. Meyer. "The Role of Glutathione in Detoxication," *Environ Health Perspect* 49 (1983): 59–69.

Leeuwenburgh, C. "Glutathione Depletion in Rested and Exercised Mice: Biochemical Consequences of Adaptation," *Arch Biochem Biophys* 316, 2 (1995): 941.

Hagen, T.M., et al. "Fate of Dietary Glutathione: Disposition in the Gastrointestinal Tract," *Am J Phys* 259, 4 (1990): G530–G535.

Dietary glutathione could be used to detoxify reactive electrophiles in the gut or can be absorbed for intracellular detoxification reactions.

Prestera, T., W. Holtzclaw, et al. "Chemical and Molecular Regulation of Enzymes That Detoxify Carcinogens," *Proc Natl Acad Sci USA* 90 (1993): 2965–69.

Davis, M., M. Wallig, et al. "In Vitro Metabolism of Cyanohydroxybutene: Formation of a Glutathione-S-transferase Catalyzed Product," *Res Commun Chem Pathol Pharmacol* 79 (1993): 343–53.

Stresser, D.M., L.F. Bjelodanes, et al. "The Anticarcinogenic 3,3 Diindolyl-methane Is an Inhibitor of Cytochrome p450. *J Biochem Toxicol* 10 (1995): 191–201; *J Biochem Toxicol* 22 (1997): 669–78.

Glycine and Detoxification

Quick, A.J. "Clinical Value of the Test for Hippuric Acid in Cases of Disease of the Liver," *Arch Intern Med* 57 (1936): 544–56.

Patel, D.K., et al. "Depletion of Plasma Glycine and the Effect of Glycine by Mouth on Salicylate Metabolism During Aspirin Overdose," *Hum Exp Toxicol* 9 (1990): 389–95.

Sugita, M., et al. "Urinary Hippuric Acid in Everyday Life," *Tokai J Exp Clin Med* 13, 4 (1988): 185–90.

Patel, D.K., et al. "Depletion of Plasma Glycine and Effect of Glycine by Mouth on Salicylate Metabolism During Aspirin Overdose," *Hum Exp Toxicol* 9 (1990): 389–95.

Levy, G. "Pharmacokinetics of Salicylate Elimination in Man," J Pharm Sci. 1965 Jul;54(7):959 67.

Healing Philosophy

Hahnemann, S. *Organon of Medicine*, 6th ed. New Delhi: Indian Books & Periodical Service, 1993.

Helicobacter Pylori

Hwang, H., et al. "Diet, Helicobacter Pylori Infection, Food Preservation, and Gastric Cancer Risk: Are There New Roles for Preventative Factors?" *Nutr Rev* 52 (1994): 72–83.

Jones, S.T.M., et al. "Chronic NSAID Use: Helicobacter Antibodies May Predict Ulcer Risk," *Br J Rheum* 30 (1991): 16–20.

Conway, C. "Truth and Consequences of Coffee," *Stanford Med* (Winter 1991): 24–26.

Correa, P. "How Does Helicobacter Pylori Infection Increase Risk of Gastric Cancer?" *Eur J Gastroenterol Hepatol* 6 (1994): 1117–18.

Bannerjee, S., et al. "Effect of Helicobacter Pylori and Its Eradication on Gastric Juice Ascorbic Acid," *Gut* 35 (1994): 317–22.

Hydrotherapy

Boyle, W., and A. Saine. *Naturopathic Hydrotherapy*. East Palestine, OH: Buckeye Naturopathic Press, 229.

Excellent review of hydrotherapy.

Thrash, A., and C. Thrash. *Home Remedies*. Seale, AL: Thrash Publications, 1981.

This important work is written by two medical doctors and is a wonderful overview of the scientific and medical research involving hydrotherapy.

Intestinal Flora

Editorial. "Intestinal Endotoxins as Mediators of Hepatic Injury: An Idea Whose Time Has Come Again," *Hepatology* 10, 5 (1989): 881–91.

Simopoulos, A.P., T. Corring, and A. Rerat, eds. "Intestinal Flora, Immunity, Nutrition and Health," *World Rev Nutr Diet* 74 (1993): 123–48.

Intestinal microflora may act either directly in toxicity or in association with endogenous metabolism of the host. The microflora could reduce toxicity of a compound or enhance toxicity. The xenobiotic metabolizing enzymes (XMEs) are found in the endoplasmic reticulum membranes of cells and are present mainly in the liver. Reactions using glutathione and glucuronic acid are the preferred pathways. Intestinal microflora can interfere with xenobiotic metabolism before or after chemical modification.

Ebringer, R.W., et al. "Sequential Studies in Ankylosing Spondylitis: Association of Klebsiella Pneumoneiae with Active Disease," *Ann Rheum Dis* 37 (1979): 145–51.

Deitch, E.A., et al. "Bacterial Translocation from the Gut Impairs Systemic Immunity," *Surgery* 109, 3 (1991): 269–76.

Spaeth, G., et al. "Food Without Fiber Promotes Bacterial Translocation from the Gut," *Surgery* 108, 2 (1990): 240–46.

Intestinal Permeability

Lipski, E. *Leaky Gut Syndrome*. New Caanan, CT: Keats Publishing, 1998.

Michi, C., et al. "Intestinal Permeability, Diet and Growth," *Lancet* 338 (1991): 1403–4.

There is an increased need for sulfur amino acids by the children with bowel permeability for hepatic detoxification of xenobiotics leaked into the portal circulation. High permeability and low urinary sulfate are associated. The more permeable the bowel, the lower the sulfate/creatine ratio.

Smith, M.D., R.A. Gibson, and P.M. Brooks. "Abnormal Bowel Permeability in Ankalosing Spondylitis and Rheumatoid Arthritis," *J Rheumatol* 18 (1985): 299–305.

Pearson, A.D., et al. "Intestinal Permeability in Children with Crohn's Disease and Celiac Disease," *Br Med J* 285 (1982): 20–21.

Intestinal permeability testing is a noninvasive way to monitor patients. Patients with bowel disease had a sixfold increase in permeability.

Jalonen, T. "Identical Intestinal Permeability Changes in Children with Different Clinical Manifestations of Cow's Milk Allergy," *J Allergy Clin Immunol* (5 November 1991): 737–42.

There are many protective factors in the intestinal mucosa intraepithelia: lymphocytes, secretory IgA, other immune globulins, mucosal coat, and microvillious membrane. Even though the milk reaction is a local event involving the complex web of protective factors, cow's milk allergy symptoms are commonly found elsewhere besides (but also including) the gut: in the respiratory tract and skin. Intestinal permeability is the best measurement for cow's milk food allergies.

Sanderson, I.R., et al. "Improvement of Abnormal Lactulose/Rhamnose Activity in Asymptomatic Patients with Crohn's Disease," *Gut* 28 (1987): 1073–76.

Shippee, R.L., et al. "Simultaneous Determination of Lactulose and Mannitol in the Urine of Burn Patients by Liquid Gas Chromatography," *Clin Chem* 36 (1992): 343–45.

Madara, J.L., et al. "Structure and Function of the Intestinal Epithelia Barrier in Health and Disease," *Br J Rheum* 9 (1990): 306–24.

Hollander, D., and H. Tarnawski. "Aging-Associated Increase in Intestinal Absorption of Macromolecules," *Gerontology* 31 (1985): 133–37.

O'Dwyer, S.T., et al. "A Single Dose of Endotoxin Increases Intestinal Permeability in Healthy Humans," *Arch Surg* 123 (1988): 1459–64.

Dietch, E.A., et al. "Bacterial Translocation from the Gut Impairs Systemic Immunity," *Surgery* 109, 3 (1991): 279–76.

Enteric bacteria and endotoxins play a role in multiple organ failure. Bacteria and their endotoxins have a major impact on the host's immune system. Bacterial translocation causes decreased systemic immune responsiveness.

Failure of the gut barrier results in further impairment of host defenses, thereby leading to increased survival of translocated bacteria.

Nolan, J.P. "Intestinal Endotoxins as Mediators of Hepatic Injury: An Idea Whose Time Has Come Again," *Hepatology* 10, 5 (1989): 887–89.

Spaeth, G., et al. "Food Without Fiber Promotes Bacterial Translocation from the Gut," *Surgery* 108, 2 (1990): 240–46.

Doctors have been treating patients for chronic disease by increasing fiber in the intestines for over one hundred years. This was one of the cornerstones of John Harvey Kellogg's work at the Battle Creek Michigan Sanitarium. Fiber helps maintain intestinal permeability.

Three things alter gut permeability: disruption of the gut flora, impaired host immune defenses, and physical disruption of the gut barrier. Once the intestinal permeability is damaged and toxins leak in, a protein-malnourished individual cannot defend itself as well.

Maintenance of gut barrier in a critically ill patient is very difficult because these patients have blood loss and are on vasoactive drugs, which could cause splanchnic vasoconstriction and gut injury. These patients also have impaired immune function because they are on antibiotics, antiulcer medications, and dietary regimens that disrupt the ecology of the flora.

The initial step of translocation is the adherence of bacteria from the intestinal tract to the epithelial cell surface or to ulcerated areas of the intestinal mucosal surface. From here they migrate across the cell surface into the circulation.

Caradonna, L., L. Amati, T. Magrone, N.M. Pellegrino, E. Jirillo, and D. Caccavo. "Enteric Bacteria, Lipopolysaccharides and Related Cytokines in Inflammatory Bowel Disease: Biological and Clinical Significance." *J Endotoxicol Res* 6, 3 (2000): 205–12.

Toxic overload in the body—triggered by increased intestinal permeability and an imbalanced microflora in the gut—may be a precipitating factor that triggers and drives inflammatory bowel disease (IBD). When the gut linings normally tight junctions become wrenched loose, increased intestinal permeability allows bacterial toxins to penetrate the gut and enter the circulation. These toxins, including dietary antigens, bacterial pathogens, toxic by-products, and bacterial cell wall lipopolysaccharides, can then ignite an intricate chain of chronic inflammatory immune reactions that damage the intestine and set off symptoms associated with IBD. As a result of this gut dysfunction, endotoxemia occurs in as many as 94 percent of patients with Crohn's disease, one of the major forms of IBD.

Intestinal Toxicity

Back, D.J., et al. "First Pass Metabolism by Intestinal Mucosa (Review)," *Aliment Pharmacol Ther* 1 (1987): 339–57.

Esterbauer, H., and H. Zollner. "Methods of Determination of Aldehyde Lipid Peroxidation Product," *Free Radic Biol Med* 7 (1989): 197–203.

Kaminsky, L.S., and M.J. Fasco. "Small Intestinal Cytochrome p450," *Crit Rev Toxicol* 1, 21 (1991): 407–22.

Iron

Salonen, J., et al. "High Stored Iron Levels Are Associated With Excess Risk of Myocardial Infarction in Eastern Finnish Men," *Circulation,* September 86(3) (1992): 803–811.

Lead

Pangborn, J. "Mechanisms of Detoxication and Procedures for Detoxification," Doctor's Data, 170 West Roosevelt Road, West Chicago, IL 60185.

Chang, L.W. *Toxicology of Metals.* Boca Raton, FL: CRC Press, 1996.

Paigen, B. "Children and Toxic Chemicals," *J Pestic Reform* 6 (1986): 2–5.

Raloff, J. "Caries: Legacy of Mom's Lead Exposure?" *Sci News* 152 (1997): 149.

Hsu, J.M. "Lead Toxicity as Related to Glutathione Metabolism," *J Nutr* 3 (1981): 26–33.

Lead Tech '92. "Proceedings and Papers from the Lead Tech 92: Solutions for a Nation at Risk", IAQ Publications, (September 1992), 4520 East West Highway, Suite 610, Bethesda , MD 20814.

Goyer, R.A., and M.G. Cherian. "Ascorbic Acid and EDTA Treatment of Lead Toxicity in Rat," *Life Sci* 24 (1979): 433–38.

Raloff, J. "New Lead Record Is No Honor," *Sci News* 154 (1998): 182.

More than 70 percent of the toddlers coming into an inner-city preschool had excess lead levels in their blood. The study was done on 817 children and excluded any children who had known lead exposure or elevated blood lead levels. Children can suffer from developmental delays, diminished IQ, small stature, and impaired balance.

Zerbino, D.D. "Chronic Effects of Lead on the Vascular System: Problem of Ecological Pathology," *APXNB* 7, 52 (1990): 70–72.

This review states that chronic lead exposure may have negative effects on the cardiovascular system. Lead toxicity eventually causes a process of vasculitis or atherosclerosis and is seen mainly in the small arteries. Every patient going through our clinic has a hair analysis to be screened for heavy metals. Chelation therapy using EDTA, DMSA, and DMPS is usually indicated in those patients who have positive hair analysis findings, especially if the findings are combined with signs of tissue and organ damage (kidney disorders, hypertension, atherosclerosis).

Moller, L., and T. Kristensen. "Blood Lead as a Cardiovascular Risk Factor," *Am J Epidemiol* 136 (1992): 1091–100.

This study supports the hypothesis that there is an association between blood lead, blood pressure, total mortality, coronary heart disease, and cardiovascular disease. The authors note that this risk for individuals appears to be very modest but for the population at large might be more significant.

Lemons

Reicks, M.M., and D. Crankshaw. "Effects of D-Limonene on Hepatic Microsomal Mono-oxygenase Activity and Paracetamol-

Induced Glutathione Depletion in a Mouse," *Xenobiotica* 23 (1993): 809–19.

Lipoic Acid

Kagen, V.E., et al. "Dihydrolipoic Acid: A Universal Antioxidant Both in the Membrane and in the Aqueous Phase," *Biochem Pharmacol* 44 (1992): 1637–49.

N-Acetyl-Cysteine

Lauterburg, B.H., et al. "Mechanism of Action of N-acetyl-cysteine in the Protection Against the Hepatotoxicity of Acetaminophen in Rats in Vivo," *J Clin Invest* 71 (1983): 980–81.

Lecithin

Duff, G.L., et al. "Lecithin, a Dietary Source of Choline, May Increase the Capacity of the Bile to Solubilize Cholesterol," *Am J Med* 11 (1951): 92.

Cowen, R. "Soybean Lecithin May Prevent Cirrhosis," *Sci News* 138 (1990): 340.

Fiber

Shah, N., et al. "Effect of Dietary Fiber Components on Fecal Nitrogen Excretion and Protein Utilization," *J Nutr* 12 (1982): 655–58.

Liver Detoxification

Brockmoller, J., and I. Roots. "Assessment of Liver Metabolic Function: Clinical Implications," *Clin Pharmacokinet Concepts* 27, 3 (1994): 216–48.

Pangborn, J. "Mechanisms of Detoxification and Procedures for Detoxification," Doctor's Data, 170 West Roosevelt Road, West Chicago, IL 60185.

Furlong, J.H. "Detoxification: A Clinical Perspective," *Q Rev Nat Med* (Fall 1997): 243–52.

PHASE 1

Kim, D.K., et al. "Inhibitory Effects of H2-Receptor Antagonists on Cytochrome P450 in Male ICR Mice," *Hum Exp Toxicol* 14 (1995): 623–29.

With a nation of people with ulcers who are on H2 receptor blocking drugs, we are slowing down their phase 1 detoxification.

Renner, E., et al. "Caffeine: A Model Compound for Measuring Liver Function," *Hepatology* 4, 1 (1984): 38–46.

Caffeine clearance is an excellent method for diagnosing subliminal disease.

Jost, G., et al. "Overnight Salivary Caffeine Clearance: A Liver Function Test Suitable for Routine Use," *Hepatology* 7, 2 (1987): 338–44.

Without this test, estimation of severity of liver disease is largely guesswork.

Anderson, K. "Dietary Regulation of Cytochrome P450," *Annu Rev Nutr* 11, 4 (1991): 141–59.

Protein increases P450, high carbohydrate reduces P450, essential fatty acids (EFA) are needed for P450, low intake of EFA lowers P450 activity, and fasting leads to decreased p450 activity, but the effect varies dramatically with different animals; some do well on it, and it enhances drug metabolism.

Guengerich, P. "Influence of Nutrients and Other Dietary Materials on Cytochrome p450 Enzymes," *Am J Clin Nutr* 61 (1995): 651S–658S.

Scavone, J.M., et al. "Differential Effect of Cigarette Smoking on Antipyrine Oxidation Versus Acetaminophen Conjugation," *Pharmacology* 40 (1990): 77–84.

Smoking induces drug oxidation rather than drug conjugation; this can cause a need for increased drug dosage. Long-term smoking can deplete conjugation stores and creates a situation of a pathological detoxifier, which is a high risk for cancer.

Liver Toxicity

Basile, A.S., et al. "Elevated Brain Concentrations of 1.4-benzodiazepenes in Fulminate Hepatic Failure," *NEJM* 325, 7 (1991): 473–78.

Hepatic encephalopathy is not an isolated disorder but a condition that has a continuum. Alterations in nervous system functioning from liver disease are underestimated in the clinical presentation of a wide variety of "toxic" disorders. Basically, the conclusion from this article is that as you get liver toxicity, you fail to break down valium-like compounds. A toxic state is truly a state of being intoxicated.

Mulle, K.D. "Benzodiazepene Compounds and Hepatic Encephalopathy," *NEJM* 325, 7 (1991): 509–11.

Someone with poor liver function fails to break down valium-like compounds. Other mechanisms of liver toxicity are (1) ammonia toxicity (correlation is poor), (2) the actions of unmetabolized multiple synergistic effects of neurotoxins (mercaptans, ammonia, fatty acids), (3) actions of false neurotransmitters, and (4) excessive GABA transmission.

Theal, R.M., and K. Scott. "Evaluating Asymptomatic Patients with Abnormal Liver Function Test Results," *Am Fam Phys* 53, 6 (1996): 2111–19.

Lee, W.M. "Drug Induced Hepatotoxicity," *NEJM* 333, 17 (1995): 1118–27.

Drug-induced liver toxicity is the complication of nearly every medication. Factors that cause damage include disruption of intracellular function, disruption of membrane integrity, indirect damage from immune medicated membrane damage, and genetic alterations in enzymes that allow the formation of harmful metabolites, competition by other drugs, and depletion of substrates required to detoxify the metabolites.

Variables affecting detoxification include age, sex, diet (minerals, caffeine, vegetable enzyme inducers, lipids, ethanol), stress, pregnancy, diabetes, hepatic disease, renal disease, immune stimuli (interferon, interleukin-6), enzyme polymorphism, drug–drug interference, and enzyme induction.

The most commonly implicated classes of drugs in liver injury are NSAIDs and antibiotics. The prognosis for patients with drug reaction liver failure is poor; mortality is 80 percent.

Medications

Ormerod, A.D., et al. "Penicillin in Milk: Its Importance in Urticaria," *Clin Allergy* 17 (1987): 229.

Letters. "Acetaminophen Poisoning and Liver Function," *NEJM* 331 (1994): 1310–12.

Alcohol disturbs the normal metabolism of acetaminophen, which then causes the reduced breakdown of the toxic metabolite NAPQI.

Brooks, A.C. "Middle Ear Infections in Children," *Sci News* (1994): 332–33.

Antibiotics don't work for otitis but are still the treatment of choice. Tubes don't work, and food allergies are known to be important, but doctors won't recommend removal of the tubes.

Buttram, H.E. "Overuse of Antibiotics and the Need for Alternatives," *Townsend Lett Doctors* (November 1991): 867–72.

There are many adverse effects of antibiotics, including:

1. Suppression of the immune system by suppressing antibody production and impairment of phagocytosis of white blood cells (Melby, K., and T. Midvelt, "Effects of Some Antibacterial Agents on the Phagocytosis of 32 P-Labeled E. coli by Human Polymorphonucleur Cells," *Acta Pathol Microbiol Scand Sect* 88 [1980]: 103–6)

2. Overgrowth of potentially harmful bacteria

3. Promotion of antibiotic resistant microorganisms

4. Promotion of Candida overgrowth

Mercury Amalgam

Summers, A.O., and S. Silverman. "Microbial Transformation of Metals," *Annu Rev Microbiol* 32 (1978): 237–72.

Summers, A.O., et al. "Mercury Released from Dental 'Silver' Fillings Provokes an Increase in Mercury and Antibiotic Resistant Bacteria in Oral and Intestinal Floras of Primates," *Antimicrob Agents Chemother* 36 (1993): 465–72.

Lorscheider, F., M. Vimy, and A. Summers. "Mercury Exposure from 'Silver' Tooth Fillings: Emerging Evidence Questions a Traditional Dental Paradigm," *FASB* 9 (1995): 504–8.

World Health Organization. *Environmental Health Criteria 118: Inorganic Mercury.* Geneva: World Health Organization, 1991.

Drasch, G., et al. "Mercury Burden of Human Fetal and Infant Tissues," *J Pediatr* 153, 8 (1994): 608–9.

Costa, M., et al. "Toxic Metals Produce an S-phase Specific Cell Cycle Block," *Res Commun Chem Pathol Pharmacol* 38 (1982): 405–19.

Ware, R., et al. "Ultrastructural Study on the Blood-Brain Barrier Dysfunction Following Mercury Intoxication," *Acta Neuropathol (Berlin)* 30 (1987): 211–24.

Nylander, M., et al. "Mercury Concentrations in Human Brain and Kidneys in Relation to Exposure from Amalgam Fillings," *Swed Dent J* 11 (1987): 179–87.

Gay, D.D., Cox RD, Reinhardt JW., et al. "Chewing Releases Mercury from Fillings," *Lancet* (1979): 985.

Schiele, R.T., et al. "Studies on the Mercury Content in Brain and Kidney Related to Number and Condition of Amalgam Fillings," Viewpoints from Medicine and Dental Medicine Symposium, Köln, Germany (1984), submitted for publication.

Gonzalez-Ramirez, D., et al. "Sodium 2,3-dimercaptopropane-1-sulfonate Challenge Test for Mercury in Humans: II. Urinary Mercury, Porphyries and Neurobehavioral Changes of Dental Workers in Monterrey, Mexico," *J Pharmacol Exp Ther* 272, 1 (1995): 264–74.

Huggins, H. "Coors Study 1997," to be published.

Katz, S.A., and R.B. Katz. "Use of Hair Analysis for Evaluating Mercury Intoxication of the Human Body: A Review," *J Appl Toxicol* 12, 2 (1992): 79–84.

Siblerud, R.L. "The Relationship Between Mercury from Dental Amalgam and Mental Health," *Am J Psychother* (18 October 1989): 575–87.

Svare, C.W., et al. "Dental Amalgam: A Potential Source of Mercury Vapor Exposure," *J Dent Res* 59, abstract 293 (1980): 341.

Vimy, M., et al. "Mercury Uptake in Sheep Fetus from Dental Fillings," paper presented at the 32nd annual meeting of the Canadian Federation of Biological Societies (June 1989).

Friberg, L., L. Kullman, et al. "Kvicksilver I Centrala Nervystement I Relation Till Amalgamfyllningar," *Lakartidningen* 83 (1986): 519–22.

Hymans, B.L., and H.C. Ballon. "Dissimilar Metals in the Mouth as a Possible Cause of Otherwise Unexplainable Symptoms," *Can Med Assoc J* 29 (1933): 488–91.

Carroll, R., et al. "Protection Against Mercuric Chloride Poisoning of the Rat Kidney," *Arzeim Forsch* 15, 2 (1965): 1361–63.

Mokranjac, M., and C. Petrovic. "Vitamin C as an Antidote in Poisoning by Fatal Doses of Mercury," *C R Hebd Seances Acad Sci* 258 (1964): 1341–42.

Methionine

Frezza, M., G. Pozzato, L. Chiesa, G. Stramentinoli, and C. Di Padova. "Reversal of Intrahepatic Cholestasis of Pregnancy in Women After High Dose S-adenosyl-L-Methionine Administration," *Hepatology* 4, 2 (1984): 274–78.

The following article summary has been modified with permission from IT Services, www.clinicalpearls.com.

Eaton, K.K., and A. Hunnisett. "Abnormalities in Essential Amino Acids in Patients with Chronic Fatigue Syndrome," *J Nutr Med* 2 (1991): 369–75.

Many amino acids were low in these chronic fatigue patients, but methionine specifically stood out as being deficient in over half the patients; phenylalanine was the next most frequent deficiency, but only in 3 out of 21 patients. A possible explanation for the low status of methionine is that it is important in the detoxifying of xenobiotics such as aromatics and organochlorines. It is also involved in antioxidant processes of free-radical scavenging. Methionine is an essential sulfur-containing amino acid in human metabolism and has three major functions: (1) As S-adenosylmethionine, it acts as a methyl group donor for a wide variety of transmethylation reactions in the body, particularly in the brain. (2) It can act as a donor of sulphydryl groups, helping in detoxification of xenobiotics in the liver. (3) It is an essential precursor of other sulfur-containing amino acids, specifically cysteine and taurine. It is also a precursor for the synthesis of the tripeptide glutathione (L-glutamyl-L-cysteinyl-glycine). These molecules play an important role in the antioxidant capacity of the body. Methionine has been known to reduce circulating histamine levels by increasing the rate of its breakdown. It is possible within the context of chronic fatigue syndrome that a significant fall in methionine concentrations may be in part responsible for the depressive and allergic aspects of the illness. Anecdotally, many chronic fatigue patients report that broad-spectrum amino acid preparations help their conditions.

Milk Thistle

Geller, L.I., L.N. Gladkikh, and M.V. Griaznova. "Treatment of Fatty Hepatosis in Diabetics," *J Probl Endokrinol* (Russia) 39 (1993): 20–22.

Reyes, H., and F.R. Simon. "Intrahepatic Cholestasis of Pregnancy: An Estrogen-Related Disease," *Semin Liver Dis* 13 (1993): 289–301.

Lang, I., K. Nekam, G. Deak, et al. "Immunomodulatory and Hepatoprotective Effects of In Vivo Treatment with Free Radical Scavengers," *Ital J Gastroenterol* 22 (1990): 283–87.

Feher, J., G. Deak, G. Muzes, et al. "Liver-Protective Action of Silymarin Therapy in Chronic Alcoholic Liver Diseases," *Orv Hetil* (Hungary) 130 (1989): 2723–27.

Salmi, H.A., and S. Sarna. "Effect of Silymarin on Chemical, Functional, and Morphological Alterations of the Liver. A Double-Blind Controlled Study," *Scand J Gastroenterol* 17 (1982): 517–21.

Magliulo, E., B. Gagliardi, and G.P. Fiori. "Results of a Double-Blind Study on the Effect of Silymarin in the Treatment of Acute Viral Hepatitis, Carried Out at Two Medical Centres," *Med Klin* (Germany) 73 (1978): 1060–65.

Muzes, G., G. Deak, I. Lang, et al. "Effect of Silimarin (Legalon) Therapy on the Antioxidant Defense Mechanism and Lipid Peroxidation in Alcoholic Liver Disease (Double-Blind Protocol). *Orv Hetil* (Hungary) 131 (1990): 863–66.

Ferenci, P., B. Dragosics, H. Dittrich, H. Frank, et al. "Randomized Controlled Trial of Silymarin Treatment in Patients with Cirrhosis of the Liver," *J Hepatol* (Netherlands) 9 (1989): 105–13.

Mind/Body Health

Mittleman, M.A., and M. Maclure. "Mental Stress During Daily Life Triggers Myocardial Ischemia," *JAMA* 277, 19 (1997): 1558–59.

Greer, S., et al. "Adjuvant Psychological Therapy for Patients with Cancer: A Prospective Randomized Trial," *Br Med J* 304 (1992): 675–80.

Spiegel, D. "Psychological Aspects of Breast Cancer Treatment," *Sem Oncol* 24, 1 (1997): S1-36–S1-47.

Goyeche, J. "Yoga as Therapy in Psychosomatic Medicine," *Psychother Psychosom* 31 (1977): 373–81.

Zojonc, R.B. "Emotion and Facial Efference: A Theory Reclaimed," *Science* 228 (1985): 15–21.

Critchly, E.M.R. "The Human Face," *Br Med J* 29 (1985): 1223–24.

Schwartz, G.E. "Biofeedback, Self-Regulation, and Patterning of Physiological Processes," *Am Sci* 63 (1975): 314–24.

Molybdenum

Rajagopalan, K.V. "Molybdenum: An Essential Element," *Nutr Rev* 45, 11 (1987): 321–28.

Multiple Chemical Sensitivity

Randolph, T.G. *Human Ecology and Susceptibility to the Chemical Environment.* Springfield, IL: Charles C. Thomas Publishers, 1962.

N-Acetyl-Cysteine

Lauterburg, B.H., et al. "Mechanism of Action of N-acetyl-cysteine in the Protection Against the Hepatotoxicity of Acetaminophen in Rats in Vivo," *J Clin Invest* 71 (1983): 980–81.

NAC boosts glutathione production and has an antitoxic effect. NAC increases sulfation slightly.

Corcoran, G.B., et al. "Effects of N-acetylcysteine on Acetaminophen Covalent Binding and Hepatic Necrosis in Mice," *J Pharmacol Exp Ther* 232, 3 (1985): 864–72.

Sulfhydryl nucleophiles like NAC act through pre-arylation mechanisms to decrease the amount of reactive metabolite available for irritation of hepatic injury.

Naturopathic Detoxification Philosophy

Boucher, J.A. "Patient Heal Thyself," *Alive: Canadian Journal of Health and Nutrition* 43 (1982): 23–24.

Neural Therapy

Dosch, P. *Manual of Neural Therapy.* Heidelberg: Haug Publishers, 1984.

Neurological Disease

Steventon, G.B., et al. "Metabolism of Low Dose Paracetamol in Patients with Chronic Neurological Disease," *Xenobiotica* 20, 1 (1990): 117–22.

Raloff, J. "Novel Antioxidants May Slow Brain's Aging," *Sci News* 151 (1997): 53.

Agid, Y. "Parkinson's Disease: Pathophysiology," *Lancet* 337 (1991): 1321–24.

Steventon, G.B. "Xenobiotic Metabolism in Parkinson's Disease," *Neurology* 39 (1989): 883–87.

Patients were found to have a reduced sulfoxidation. Poor sulfation and sulfoxidation have been found in patients with motor neuron disease. In humans, 95 percent of dopamine is sulfate-conjugated, and the biochemical consequences of this are that this pathway can become saturated, possibly due to inadequate sulfate supply. This metabolic defect may put these patients at risk for exposure to environmental or endogenous compounds. Cysteine dioxygenase from poor sulfoxidation could deposit basal ganglia iron, the same as is found in Parkinson's disease, since the thiol group acts as a metal chelator, which could lead to free-radical formation, accumulation, and cellular damage.

Heafield, M.T., et al. "Plasma Cysteine and Sulphate Levels in Patients with Motor Neuron, Parkinson's and Alzheimer's Disease," *Neurosci Lett* 110 (1990): 216–20.

Sullivan, K. "The Evidence Linking Silver-Mercury Fillings to Alzheimer's Disease: Literature Review," *Townsend Lett Doctors* (August 1997): 74–83.

Davis, K.L., and J.A. Yesavage. *Brain Acetylcholine and Neuropsychiatric Disease.* New York: Plenum Press, 1978, 205.

Hadijivassiliou, M. "Does Cryptic Gluten Sensitivity Play a Part in Neurologic Illness?" *Lancet* 347 (1996): 369–71.

Nutrition

Beasley, J.D., and J.J. Swift. *The Kellogg Report.* Annandale-on-Hudson, NY: The Institute of Health Policy and Practice, 1989.

Bland, J. *Medical Applications of Clinical Nutrition.* New Caanan, CT: Keats Publishing, 1983.

Organ Prolapse

Barral, J.P., and P. Mercier. *Visceral Manipulation*. Seattle, WA: Eastland Press, 1988.

Orthomolecular Medicine

Pauling, L., and M. Rath. "An Orthomolecular Theory of Human Health and Disease," *J Orthomol Med* 6, 3–4 (1991): 135–38.

Hoffer, A. *Orthomolecular Medicine for Physicians*. New Caanan, CT: Keats Publishing, 1989.

Definitive review of the use of vitamins and minerals in the treatment of disease and psychiatric disorders.

Pancreatitis

Braganza, J.M., J.E. Jolley, et al. "Occupational Chemicals and Pancreatitis: A Link?" *Int J Pancreatol* 1 (1986): 9–19.

Pantothenic Acid

Ellestad-Sayed, J.J., et al. "Pantothenic Acid, Coenzyme A and Human Chronic Ulcerative and Granulomatous Colitis," *Am J Clin Nutr* 29 (1976): 1333–38.

Colonic mucosa concentrates B_5 at 50 times the level of blood. Colitis patients had very low CoA in colonic mucosa.

Pesticides

Liang, H. "Clinical Evaluation of the Poisoned Patient and Toxic Syndromes," *Clin Chem* 42, 8B (1996): 1350–55.

Organophosphate and carbamates are among the most common classes of pesticides in agricultural and household settings. Poisoning is devastating because of the irreversible binding and inactivation of choline esterase. Cholinesterase inhibitors allow accumulation of acetylcholine in the central and peripheral nervous synapses. Accumulation of acetylcholine stimulates (but soon paralyzes) conduction through cholinergic synapses in the central nervous system, parasympathetic terminals, some sympathetic terminals (muscarinic), somatic nerves, and autonomic ganglionic synapses (nicotinic) .

Steingraber, S. *Living Downstream: An Ecologist Looks at Cancer and the Environment.* Reading, MA: Addison-Wesley, 1997.

Westin, J.B., and E. Richter. "The Israeli Breast Cancer Anomaly," *Ann NY Acad Sci* 609 (1990): 269–79.

Olson, L. "The Immune System and Pesticides," *J Pestic Reform* 6 (1986): 20–25.

Duffy, F.H. "Long-Term Effects of the Organophosphate Sarin on EEGs in Monkeys and Humans," *Neurotoxicity* 1 (1980): 667–89.

Yound, B.B. "Neurotoxicity of Pesticides," *J Pestic Reform* 6 (1986): 8–12.

Blair, A. "Herbicides and Non-Hodgkins Lymphoma: New Evidence from a Study of Saskatchewan Farmers," *J Int Cancer Inst* 85 (1990): 544–45.

U.S. Environmental Protection Agancy. "Respondents Brief. Proposed Findings and Conclusion on Suspension. Consolidated Aldrin-Dieldrin Hearings." FIFRA Dockets 145 (26 September 1974): 109.

Epstein, S.S. "The Carcingenicity of Organochlorine Pesticides," in H.H. Hiatt, J.D. Watson, and J.A. Winston, eds. *Origins of Human Cancer, Vol 4.* Cold Spring Harbor, NY: Cold Spring Harbor Laboratory, 1977, 243–65.

Raloff, J. "The Pesticide Shuffle," *Sci News* 149 (1996): 174–175.

United States manufacturers continue to ship DDT to third-world countries. Data are now showing that these chemicals, when used in warm tropical countries, go into the atmosphere and then condense in cooler northern climates.

Rice

Helm, R.M., and A.W. Burks. "Hypoallergenicity of Rice Protein," *Cereal Foods World* 41 (1996): 839–43.

Graf, E. "Antioxidant Potential of Ferulic Acid," *Free Radic Biol Med* 13 (1992): 435–48.

Pizarro, D., et al. "Rice-Based Oral Electrolyte Solutions for the Management of Infantile Diarrhea," *NEJM* 324 (1991): 517–21.

Solutions based on rice reduce stool output as well as restore fluid volume. Glucose solutions do not reduce the severity of the diarrhea. Rice syrup solids are effective in rehydration of infants with acute diarrhea. They decrease stool output and promote greater absorption and retention of fluid and electrolytes than glucose-based products.

Wong, H.B. "Rice Water in Treatment of Infant Gastroenteritis," *Lancet* 2, 82310 (1981): 102–3.

Wanatabe, M., et al. "Production of Hypo-Allergenic Rice by Enzymatic Decomposition of Constituent Proteins," *J Food Sci* 55, 3 (1990): 781–83.

Sulfation/Sulfoxidation

Oguro, T., et al. "Molybdate Depletes Hepatic 3-phosphoadenosie 5-phosphosulfate and Impairs the Sulfation of Acetaminophen in Rats," *J Pharmacol Exp Ther* 270 (1994): 1145–51.

Molybdenum is important for flavoprotein enzymes. Molybdate competes with sulfate in the first step from sulfate to PAPS and inhibits biosynthesis.

Levy, G. "Sulfate Conjugation in Drug Metabolism: Role of Inorganic Sulfate," *FASEB* 45 (1986): 2235–40.

Sulfation is important for biotransformation of amine neurotransmitters, steroid hormones, drugs, xenobiotics, and phenolics. The body gets rid of phenolics by glucuronidation and sulfation. The availability of sulfate in the central nervous system may modify certain neurotransmitters and other endogenous substances that are subject to sulfate metabolism. Systemic depletion of inorganic sulfate secondary to the utilization for the sulfation of drugs affects the internal environment.

Brat, R., and J.D. Beckman. "Inhibition of Phenolsulfotransferase by Pyridoxal Phosphate" *Biochem Pharmacol* 47 (1994): 2087–95.

Emery, P., et al. "D-Penicillamine Induced Toxicity in Rheumatoid Arthritis: The Role of Sulfoxidation Status and HLA-DR3," *J Rheum* 11, 5 (1984): 626–32.

Scadding, G.K., et al. "Poor Sulfoxidation Ability in Patients with Food Sensitivity," *Br Med J* 297 (1988): 105–7.

Sulfoxidation is the process by which sulfur-containing molecules in drugs and foods are metabolized. It is also the process by which sulfites are eliminated. Food reactions run in families. Seventy-eight percent of 74 patients were poor sulfoxidizers. There was a greater prevalence of poor sulfoxidizers among patients whose symptoms were exacerbated by certain foods. Foods contain numerous xenobiotics containing sulfur, thiophenes, sulfides, and isothiocyanates, which undergo metabolic oxidation in the body. Sulfoxidation state may reflect the patient's ability to provide sulfate precursors for conjugation by means of intermediary metabolism. A limited sulfation ability leaves immunogenic chemical groups free to mediate various allergic responses.

Synergy of Toxins

Schubert, J., et al. "Synergistic Effects of Lead and Mercury," *J Toxicol Environ Health* 4 (1978): 763–76.

Abou-Donia, et al. "Neurotoxicity Resulting from Coexposure to Pyristigmine Bromide, DEET and Permethrin: Implications of Gulf War Exposures," *J Toxicol Environ Health* 48 (1996): 35–56.

Raloff, J. "'Estrogen' Pairings Can Increase Potency," *Sci News* 149 (1996): 356.

A pair of PCBs have 20 times the capacity to switch the sex of animals than when given each separately. When endosulfan and dieldrin are combined, they deliver 1,600 times the effect of the dieldrin alone. Combining estrogen-mimicking agents represents compelling reasons to evaluate the use of pesticides in the food chain.

Null, G. "Immune Augmentation Therapy for Gulf War Syndrome," *Townsend Lett Doctors Patients* (April 1998): 54–58.

Excellent review of the multiple chemical exposure that happened to army personnel during the war and the aftereffects.

Sacchromyces Boulardii

Caetano, J.A., et al. "Immunopharmacological Effects of Sacchromyces Boulardii in Healthy Human Volunteers," *Int J Immunopharmacol* 8 (1986): 245–59.

Sauna

Winterfield, H.J., et al. "The Use of Walking and Sauna Therapy in the Rehabilitation of Hypertensive Patients with Ischemic Heart Disease Following Aortocoronary Venous Bypass Operation with Special Reference to Hemodynamics," *Z Kardiol* 77 (1988): 190–93.

Winterfield, H.J., et al. "Sauna Therapy in Coronary Heart Disease with Hypertension After Bypass Operation in Heart Aneurysm Operation and in Essential Hypertension," *Z Gesamte Inn Med* 48 (1993): 247–50.

Parpalei, P.A., et al. "The Use of Sauna for Disease Prevention in the Workers of Enterprises with Chemical and Physical Occupational Hazards," *Vrach Delo* 5 (1991): 93–95.

Cohn, J.R., and E.A. Emmett. "The Excretion of Trace Metals in Human Sweat," *Ann Clin Lab Sci* 8 (1989): 270–75.

Arner, P. "Differences in Lipolysis Between Human Subcutaneous and Omental Adipose Tissues," *Ann Med* 27 (1995): 435–38.

Berlan, M., et al. "Lipid Mobilization, Physiopathological and Pharmocological Aspects," *Ann Endocrinol* 56 (1995): 97–100.

Cession-Fossion, A., et al. "Influence of Sauna Baths on Urinary Excretion of Catecholamines," *C R Sceances Soc Biol Fil* 171 (1977): 1313–16.

Hussi, E., et al. "Plasma Catecholamines in Finnish Sauna," *Ann Clin Res* 9 (1977): 301–4.

Lammintausta, R., et al. "Change in Hormones Reflecting Sympathetic Activity in the Finnish Sauna," *Ann Clin Res* 8 (1976): 266–71.

Omokhodion, F.O., and J.M. Howard. "Trace Elements in the Sweat of Acclimatized Persons," *Clin Chem Acta* 231 (1994): 23–28.

Press, E. "The Health Hazards of Saunas and Spas and How to Minimize Them," *Am J Pub Health* 81 (1991): 10434–37.

Kilburn, K.H., et al. "Neurobehavioural Dysfunction in Firemen Exposed to Polychlorinated Biphenyls (PCBs): Possible Improvement After Detoxification." *Arch Int Health* 44, 9 (1989): 345–49.

Schnare, D.W., et al. "Evaluation of a Detoxification Regimen for Fat Stored Xenobiotics," *Med Hypotheses* 9 (1982): 265–82.

Review of a Hubbard detoxification protocol for the purpose of those exposed to xenobiotics

Program for three weeks' duration: physical exercise for 20 to 30 minutes; 140- to 180-degree-Fahrenheit sauna for two and a half hours; vitamin C, A, D, E, B complex; minerals Ca, Mg, Fe, Zn, Mg, Cu, K, I; essential fatty acids.

Selenium

Anderson, O., and J.B. Neilson. "Effects of Simultaneous Low Level Dietary Supplementation with Inorganic and Organic Selenium on Whole Body Blood and Organ Levels of Toxic Metals in Mice," *Environ Health Perspect* 102, Suppl. 3 (1994): 321–24.

Neve, J. "Physiologic and Nutritional Importance of Selenium," *Experientia* 47 (1991): 187–93. Reviewed by Kirk Hamilton, with permission from IT Services, www.clinicalpearls.com.

Selenium is important because it is used in the detoxification enzyme glutathione peroxidase. Current research has shown selenium to be effective in the prevention of degenerative free-radical disease such as neurologic diseases, inflammatory diseases, and cancer. In Africa selenium deficiency is involved in neurologic disturbances in conjunction with iodine deficiency. Hemolytic anemia and immune dysfunction are also signs of selenium deficiency. Selenium deficiency has been associated with neuronal ceroid lipofuscinosis and encephalopathy, caused by accumulation in the central nervous system of lipid peroxide products. Down's syndrome patients have increased glutathione peroxidase activity resulting in rapid aging and cerebral degeneration. In alcoholic cirrhosis, blood and liver selenium levels are low in addition to increased peroxidative liver damage. Decreased selenium has been related to increased prothrombin time. Low selenium levels have been significantly associated with the number of affected joints and mobility in rheumatoid arthritic patients. Doses vary widely around the world. One hundred and fifty to 300 mcg per day of selenium have been used to prevent Keshan's cardiomyopathy in China. In low-soil-selenium populations such as Finland or Denmark, selenium supplements are given to the population by adding it to animal feed or fertilizers. Supplementation with 100 to 150 mcg per day of selenium has benefited some rheumatoid arthritic patients. Selenium deficiency is also associated with cystic fibrosis. Increased lipid peroxidation may result in pulmonary problems. In renal-insufficiency patients on dialysis, there is an inverse relationship between peroxidation products and blood selenium levels.

Peroxidation is also seen in the muscular dystrophies and myotonic dystrophy; treatment with selenium and vitamin E supplementation in these conditions has shown benefit. There has been shown a positive relationship between plasma selenium and left-ventricular function in nonobstructive cardiomyopathies. Inverse correlations have been seen between low plasma selenium levels and the severity of atherosclerosis. A relationship has also been seen between selenium and HDL cholesterol. Low plasma selenium, less than 45μ selenium per liter, has been considered a significant risk factor in Finland for cardiovascular disease. Selenium is a potent anticarcinogenic agent. Epidemiologic studies support its role as a chemopreventive agent. Selenium supplementation has shown benefit in preventing hepatitis B–induced liver cancer, and several hundred mcg per day of this element can serve as an adjunctive treatment for breast cancer.

Stress and Detoxification

Bernton, E., D. Hoover, R. Galloway, and K. Popp. "Adaptation to Chronic Stress in Military Trainees," *Ann NY Acad Sci* 774 (1995): 217–31.

A very revealing article that makes the connection between stress, insulin resistance, and detoxification. Chinese doctors described poor liver detoxification from stress over a thousand years ago. We usually think that the detoxification enzyme system reacts as a consequence of exposure to exobiotics or alteration in hormone levels including progesterone, estrogen, and thyroxin. This study shows that stress can also cause a toxic reaction by altering the p450 gene as a result of the secretion of glucocorticoids.

Findings: Increased free salivary cortisol levels, decreased testosterone-to-hypogonadal levels, increased salivary DHEA, insulin insensitivity, and increased gut permeability (stress is literally toxic).

Conclusion: High levels of cortisol cause the full expression of the gene to regulate P4501A1 synthesis. This could result in the significant increases in carcinogenic risk as a consequence of enhanced conversion of procarcinogens (bottle neck detoxification) with this enzyme to intermediary carcinogens.

Matthews, S.B., et al. "The Adrenochrome Pathway: The Major Route for Adrenalin Catabolism by Polymorphonuclear Cells," *J Mol Cell Cardiol* 17 (1985): 339–48.

Dhalla, K.S., et al. "Measurement of Adrenolurin as an Oxidation Product of Catecholamine in Plasma," *Mol Cell Biochem* 87 (1989): 85–92.

James, R.C., et al. "Phenylpropanolamine Potentiation of Acetaminophen-Induced Hepatotoxicity: Evidence for a Glutathione-Dependent Mechanism," *Toxicol App Pharmacol* 118 (1993): 159–68.

Adrenergic stimulation (stress-induced adrenalin production) depresses glutathione to the extent that it can cause acetaminophen toxicity. Mechanism is not known.

Vergano, D. "Stress May Weaken the Blood Brain Barrier," *Sci News* 150 (1996): 375.

Mittleman, M.A., M. Maclure, and Editorial. "Mental Stress During Daily Life Triggers Myocardial Ischemia," *JAMA* 277, 19 (1997): 1558–59.

Schnall, P.L., et al. "The Relationship Between 'Job Strain' Workplace Diastolic Blood Pressure, and Left Ventricular Mass Index: Results of a Case Controlled Study," *JAMA* 263, 14 (1990): 1929–35.

Systems Theory and Medicine

Davidson, M. *Uncommon Sense: The Life and Thought of Ludwig von Bertalanffy, Father of General Systems Theory.* Los Angeles, CA: J.P. Tarcher, 1983, 27.

Taurine

Yamanaka, Y., et al. "Effects of Dietary Taurine on Cholesterol Gallstone Formation," *J Nutr Sci Vitaminol* (1985): 31–32.

Turmeric

Roa, S. "Nitric Oxide Scavenging by Curcuminoids," *J Pharm Pharmacol* 49 (1997): 105–7.

Vegetables

Nijihoff, W.A., M.J. Grubben, et al. "Effects of Consumption of Brussels Sprout on Intestinal and Lymphocytic Glutathione S-transferases in Humans," *Carcinogenesis* 16 (1995): 2125–28.

Stresser, D.M., L.F. Bjelodanes, et al. "The Anticarcinogenic 3,3 Diindolyl-methane Is an Inhibitor of Cytochrome p450," *J Biochem Toxicol* 10 (1995): 191–201.

Vitamin C

Riordan, N.H., H.D. Riordan, et al. "Intravenous Ascorbate as a Tumor Cytotoxic Chemotherapeutic Agent," *Med Hypotheses* 44 (1995): 207–13.

The research of Dr. Hugh Riordan has shown that in high intravenous doses, vitamin C can be toxic to cancer tumors. Vitamin C therapy was originally pioneered by Dr. Fredrick Klenner in the 1950s. He showed that vitamin C in intravenous doses could treat cancer as well as prevent the fatal effects of many serious diseases such as viral meningitis, insect stings, and polio. Many physicians have reproduced Dr. Klenner's studies with similar findings.

Goyer, R.A., and M.G. Cherian. "Ascorbic Acid and EDTA Treatment of Lead Toxicity in Rats. *Life Sci* 24 (1979): 433–38.

Carroll, R., et al. "Protection Against Mercuric Chloride Poisoning of the Rat Kidney," *Arzeim Forsch* 15, 2 (November 1965): 1361–63.

Vauthey, M. "Protective Effect of Vitamin C Against Poisons," *Praxis* 40 (1951): 284–86.

Murray, D.R., and R.E. Hughes. "The Influence of Dietary Ascorbic Acid on the Concentration of Mercury in Guinea Pig Tissues," *Proc Nutr Sci* 35 (1976): 118–19.

Hill, C.H. "Studies on the Ameliorating Effect of Ascorbic Acid on Mineral Toxicities in the Chick," *J Nutr* 109, 1 (1979): 84–90.

Gupta, G.C., and B.C. Guha. "The Effect of Vitamin C and Certain Other Substances on the Growth of Microorganisms," *Ann Biochem Exp Med* 1 (1941): 14–26.

Sirsi, M. "Antimicrobial Action of Vitamin C on M Tuberculosis and Some Other Pathogenic Organisms," *Indian J Med Sci* 6 (1952): 252–55.

Jungeblut, C.W. "Inactivation of Tetanus Toxin by Crystalline Vitamin C (Ascorbic Acid)," *J Immunol* 33 (1937): 203–14.

Jungeblut, C.W., and R.L. Swemer. "Inactivation of Diphtheria Toxin in Vivo and in Vitro by Crystalline Vitamin C (Ascorbic Acid)," *Proc Soc Exp Biol Med* 32 (1935): 1229–34.

Kodama, T., and T. Kojina. "Studies of the Staphylococcal Toxin, Toxoid and Antitoxin: Effect of Ascorbic Acid on Staphylococcal Lysins and Organisms," *Kitasato Arch Exp Med* 16 (1939): 36–35.

Perdomo, J.H. "Snake Venom and Vitamin C," *Rev Fac Med (Bogota)* 15 (1947): 769–72.

Frossman, S., and Frykholm, KO. "Benzene Poisoning II," *Acta Med Scand* 128 (1947): 256–80.

Dey, P.K. "Protection Action of Ascorbic Acid and Its Precursors on the Convulsive and Lethal Actions of Strychnine," *Indian J Exp Biol* 5 (1967): 110–12.

Vitamin C Safety

KIDNEY STONES

Chalmers, A.H., et al. "Stability of Ascorbate in Urine: Relevance to Analyses for Ascorbate and Oxalate," *Clin Chem* 31 (1985): 1703.

Wandzilak, T.R., et al. "Effect of High Dose Vitamin C on Urinary Oxalate Levels," *J Urol* 151 (1994): 834–37.

HEMOLYSIS

Chiu, D.T., et al. "Blood Vitamin C in Human Glucose-6-phosphate Dehydrogenase Deficiency. Vitamin C." *Health Dis* (1997): 323–31.

A 1975 paper, based on anecdotal evidence, reported that vitamin C induced the destruction of red blood cells (hemolysis) when given to individuals with a genetic enzyme deficiency called G-6-PD. This enzyme deficiency affects 200 million people worldwide and causes such symptoms as neonatal jaundice and hemolytic anemia. Some physicians recommended having a test that would determine if a patient had this problem before recommending high doses of vitamin C.

In 1997, however, the above paper was published, which showed that patients with G-6-PD had very low levels of vitamin C in their blood, suggesting that those with this disease need extra vitamin C and other antioxidants. Low levels of vitamin C in these patients may actually put them at risk for the condition.

Vitamin E

Sword, J.T., et al. "Endotoxin and Lipid Peroxidation in Vivo in Selenium and Vitamin E Deficient and Adequate Rats," *J Nutr* 121 (1991): 258–64.

Packer, L. "Vitamin E Is Nature's Master Antioxidant," *Scientific American* (March/April 1994): 54–63.

Esterbauer, H., and H. Zollner. "Methods of Determination of Aldehyde Lipid Peroxidation Product," *Free Radic Biol Med* 7 (1989): 197–203.

Raloff, J. "Vitamin E Helps—but Don't Overdose," *Sci News* 151 (1997): 135.

Vitamin A

Cullum, M.E., and M.H. Zile. "Acute Polybrominated Biphenyl Toxicosis Alters Vitamin A Homeostasis and Enhances Degradation of Vitamin A. *Toxicol Appl Pharmacol* 81 (1985): 177–81.

RECOMMENDED READING

Nutritional Medicine

Murray, M. *Encyclopedia of Nutritional Supplements.* Rocklin, CA: Prima Publishing, 1996.

Price, W. *Nutrition and Physical Degeneration,* 6th ed. New Caanan, CT: Keats Publishing, 1997.

Werbach, M. *Nutritional Influences on Illness,* 2nd ed. Tarzana, CA: Third Line Press, 1993.

Naturopathic Medicine

Boyle W., and F. Kirchefeld. *Nature Doctors.* East Palestine: OH: Buckeye Press, 1995.

Pizzorno J.P., and M. Murray. *Encyclopedia of Natural Medicine.* Rocklin, CA: Prima Publishing, 1990.

Detoxification Medicine

MacDonald, S.M. *Detoxification and Healing.* New Caanan, CT: Keats Publishing, 1997.

Rauch, E. *Health Through Inner Body Cleansing.* Brussels: International, 1993.

Rogers, S. *Tired or Toxic.* Syracuse, NY: Prestige Publishing, 1990.

Hydrotherapy

Boyle W., and A. Saine. *Lectures in Naturopathic Hydrotherapy.* East Palestine, OH: Buckeye Naturopathic Press, 1988.

Buchman, D. *The Complete Book of Water Therapy.* New Caanan, CT: Keats Publishing, 1994

Thrash A., and C. Thrash. *Home Remedies.* Seale, AL: Thrash Publications, 1981.

INDEX

Self-deprecation/self-destruction, 10
Self-hypnosis, 93, 231
Sensory system, 37
Serotonin, 218, 308
Sesame Rice Casserole, 248
Setting for eating, 268
Seven-day EcoTox program. *See* EcoTox
    program
Seven-day schedule sample, 281–297
SGOT (serum glutamic oxaloacetic
    transaminase) test, 140
SGPT (serum glutamic pyruvic transami-
    nase), 140–141
Shale oil, 120
Shavasana, 230–231
Shaw, Bill, 160
Shower method hydrotherapy, 220–221
Silent Spring, The, 29
Silymarin, 208–209
Sinus infections, 171
Sinusitis, 83
Skepticism about EcoTox program, 258–259
Skin. *See also* Sweat therapy
    dry skin brushing, 225–226
    elimination of toxins, 80–81
    healthy skin, 45–46
    pesticides and cancer, 129
    stress and, 10
    toxicity symptoms, 37
    zinc deficiency and, 212
Sleep disorders
    amino acid conversion and, 161
    DHEA and, 162
    EcoTox program and, 185
    melatonin levels, testing, 163
Smart Fats, 61
Smell of foods, 266
Smoking. *See* Cigarette smoking
Smoothies, 250
Snacks
    Hummus, 251
    Rice Cakes and Guacamole, 252
Snake venom, 193
Sodium, 147
Soft drinks, 103
Solvents, 105, 107
Soups
    Bieler broth, 240
    Borscht, 241
    Miso soup, 240–241
    Mung soup, 241
South America, mercury poisoning in, 134
Sperm, 135
Spinach Tofu Quiche, 246–247
Stale foods, 127
Standard of care model, 25
Staph infections, 193
Stasis of blood, 73
Steam baths, 225
Steaming vegetables, 242
Steingraber, Sandra, 128
Steroids, 93

bacterial equilibrium and, 205
detoxification treatment and, 14
gastrointestinal (GI) system and, 83
pantothenic acid and, 210
Phase 1 detoxification and, 104
probiotics with, 206
sulfation and, 102
Stillbirth, mercury and, 135
Stir fry vegetables, 242
Stomach, 129
Stool, 78–80, 152–154
Stress
    disease and, 10
    hormones, 10
    mind training and, 227–228
    transforming, 90–93
Stretching, 67
String Beans with Marinade, 243
Strychnine, 193
Styrene, 119
Sugars. *See* Glucose
Sulfation, 102
    genetics and, 114
Sulfhydryl protein, 59
Sulfites, 211, 212
Sulfonamide medications, 104
Sulfoxidation
    methionine and, 200–201
    symptoms of, 201
Sulfur, 102, 147
Sunflower, 183
Superoxide dismutase, 211–212
Sweat therapy, 3, 77, 223–225
    benefits of, 81–82
    circulation, improving, 223–225
    water intake and, 80
Sympathetic nervous system
    alternate-nostril breathing, 229
    circulation and, 73–74
    disorders of, 74
Synergy, 27–30

T
Tahini Sauce, 246
Taraxacum, 112, 201
Taste of foods, 266–267
Taurine, 102, 112, 200
Teas
    Fruit Tea, 253
    green tea, 208
Teeth. *See* Dentistry
Temperature of foods, 267
Terminal/malignant illnesses, 170
Tetanus, 193
Thiazide diuretics, 141
Thirst and hunger, 173
Tilden, John H., 166
Time considerations, 259–260
Tofu
    Creamy Tofu Dressing, 244
    Spinach Tofu Quiche, 246–247

ABOUT THE AUTHORS

Peter Bennett, N.D., is medical director of Helios Clinic in Victoria, British Columbia, where he supervises the care of patients in the Ecotox detoxification and Lifetime Performance wellness programs. He graduated with a doctorate in naturopathic medicine from Bastyr University. Dr. Bennett uses hydrotherapy, diet, and intravenous nutritional medicines to help patients with acute and chronic health problems. As a board-certified acupuncturist and homeopathic practitioner, he works with his patients using a program of holistic care. He frequently lectures to the public and health care professionals, writes for magazines, and has been a featured expert on national television programs.

Stephen Barrie, N.D., is the founder and president of Great Smokies Diagnostic Laboratory, a leader in functional medicine testing for physicians throughout the world. A naturopathic physician who graduated from Bastyr University, Dr. Barrie has written for numerous medical journals and lectured on detoxification and gastrointestinal health at medical conferences worldwide. He lives in Asheville, North Carolina.

Sara Faye is an award-winning freelance journalist and author. She has been writing about health and medicine for more than twenty-five years. While working with Drs. Bennett and Barrie on *7-Day Detox Miracle,* she followed the detoxification program and discovered its value firsthand.